Dr Val Wilson holds a PhD in Health Education from the University of Kent. Her thesis concerned effective self-management of diabetes. She also holds an MSc in Health Education and Health Promotion from Canterbury Christ Church University. Dr Wilson has published widely in nursing and healthcare journals, and has had Type 1 diabetes for forty-three years.

How to Reduce Your Child's Sugar Intake

A Quick and Easy Guide to Improving
Your Family's Health

••••••••••••••••••••

Val Wilson

A How To book

ROBINSON

ROBINSON

First published in Great Britain in 2021 by
Robinson

10 9 8 7 6 5 4 3 2 1

Important Note
The recommendations in this book are
solely intended as education and
information and should not be taken as
medical advice.

A CIP catalogue record for this book
is available from the British Library.

ISBN: 978-1-47214-489-8

Typeset in Sentinel and Scala Sans
by Ian Hughes

Printed and bound in Great Britain by Clays
Ltd, Elcograf S.p.A.

Papers used by Robinson are from well-
managed forests and other responsible
sources.

MIX
Paper from
responsible sources
FSC® C104740

Robinson
An imprint of
Little, Brown Book Group
Carmelite House
50 Victoria Embankment
London EC4Y 0DZ

An Hachette UK Company
www.hachette.co.uk

www.littlebrown.co.uk

How To Books are published by
Robinson, an imprint of Little, Brown
Book Group. We welcome proposals
from authors who have first-hand
experience of their subjects. Please set
out the aims of your book, its target
market and its suggested contents in an
email to howto@littlebrown.co.uk.

For Neil

Contents

Introduction

As someone who has had Type 1 diabetes for forty-three years, I have a very unhealthy relationship with sugar. Sugar is as addictive as nicotine and because our bodies aren't designed to cope with it, reducing sugar intake – especially for children – is a must. Sugar triggers the release of dopamine in the brain, the same 'pleasure' response that stimulants such as nicotine and caffeine also trigger. Due to the way sugar enhances pleasure receptors, the enjoyment derived from eating something sweet becomes addictive. A news report in January 2019 stated that children will have 'eaten twenty stones of sugar by age ten'[1] – that's 280 pounds or 127kg of sugar in the first ten years of a child's life.

We know what the average sugar consumption is in each country, but it is difficult to find answers to simple questions like how much sugar is eaten by people of different ages, or what is the average sugar content in the diet of eleven-year-old British schoolchildren. There is no physiological requirement for sugar in our diets; all human nutrition needs can be fully met without having to consume even a spoonful of any kind of sugar, or sugars added by manufacturers to our food and drink. In a diabetic diet, the emphasis is on keeping blood glucose levels stable to manage the condition as well as possible, and this is something I discuss comprehensively in my book *How to Live Well with Diabetes*. However, it's not just people with diabetes who need to be wary of eating a high-sugar diet – the same goes for everyone else too.

We all have a hard wired attraction to sweet things as a protection measure; poisonous berries are sour-tasting and dangerous, so sweet things taste much better. Eating habits are formed in early childhood and children undoubtedly like sweet foods, even though they are not healthy foods. In 1715 Dr Frederick Slare, an important member of the College of Physicians and supporter of the sugar industry, observed how children positively react to sugar: 'Give babies a choice of sugar water or plain, and they will greedily suck down the one, and make faces at the other: Nor will they be pleased with cow's milk, unless that be blessed with a little sugar, to bring it up to the sweetness of breast milk.'[2]

Unfortunately, modern society tends to revolve around treats, rewards and celebrations where mostly high-sugar foods are on offer: cinema visits, where you can buy sweets, chocolates and sugary popcorn by the bucketful; vending machines, petrol stations and newsagents selling high-sugar fizzy drinks; birthdays celebrated with cake covered in thick, sweet icing, frosting or ganache made with powdered sugar; Easter eggs; Halloween, when the focus for children is on getting a big haul of sweets and chocolate bars; and Christmas with its 'traditional' cake, pudding, mince pies, sweets and chocolates – the list is endless. This means we are now surrounded by sugar.

In recent times, the relationship between high-sugar foods and ill health has worryingly been highlighted in the news. From Type 2 diabetes occurring in obese children as young as three years old to hyperactivity and poor dental health, the over-consumption of sweet foods and drinks by children and young adults has created a significant health time bomb. One-third of primary-school children are now classed as overweight or obese and one-quarter of five-year-olds has significant tooth decay, both conditions being due to excess sugar consumption. Children who are overweight are likely to remain that way into adulthood, increasing their risk of developing Type 2 diabetes, heart disease and certain cancers. These problems suggest that the amount of dietary sugar should be reduced.

A child's behaviour and emotional health – mood swings, temper tantrums, inability to concentrate and lack of energy – are not a result of them choosing to be difficult, but are often influenced by the way sugar in the diet affects brain chemistry. Children are more sensitive than adults to blood glucose fluctuations. Rapidly altering blood glucose levels can be caused by irregular mealtimes, eating lots of refined carbohydrates with a high sugar content and not getting the nutrients required. Erratic blood glucose levels may cause children to become moody, unpredictable, light-headed or energetic and easily distracted. This book will explain why your child can suddenly change personality and how to address this situation permanently by getting to the root of the problem.

Why sugar is an issue

Since man began to produce food instead of hunting and gathering, the human diet has contained large amounts of carbohydrates of one sort or another. People were consuming carbohydrates by eating starch from wheat, rice or maize whenever they could. It was hailed as an advancement when this bland diet was enhanced with the luxury of sugar for those that could afford it; sugar became the must-have commodity. By the middle of the sixteenth century sugar, known as white gold, was as expensive as caviar and by the eighteenth century it was still regarded as a luxury. From this point on, simple starches have gradually been replaced in our diets by a greater consumption of sugar. The cost of sugar is now far less than it once was, but even 100 years ago, sugar was kept in the home in locked boxes because it was so precious. As the production process became more efficient the cost of sugar became cheaper, and as a result the consumption of sugar increased dramatically.

By the mid-1940s sugar formed one-quarter of the foods we ate; it now forms a staggering three-quarters of our diet.[3] With the introduction of sweetened drinks and confectionery at the end of the 1960s, the average person in the UK was consuming 54kg (120lb) of sugar per year; sugary breakfast cereals, soft drinks and fruit juice being responsible for this huge increase. Humans have always enjoyed eating fruit and honey because of the sweet taste but this hunger for pleasure can now be satiated with manufactured foods and drinks that are full of calories but no nutrition. The availability of such high-sugar consumables has led to a state of 'malnutrition of affluence', a term first coined by Professor John Yudkin in 1972.[4] Consumption of sugar has now decreased marginally due to the widespread use of artificial sweeteners in soft drinks, but intake is still excessive as manufacturers add sugar to more and more foods.

Today, in the West, we consume on average twenty times more sugar than our ancestors did 300–400 years before, and even the amount of sugar they ate was far greater than our ancient ancestors ever consumed due to the advent of manufacturing. Recent research suggests that sugar has a unique effect on the body, being distinctly different to that of carbohydrates like bread, potatoes and pasta. Since sugar now amounts to one-tenth of the daily calories consumed in wealthy countries, it is essential that more is known about the effect sugar has when it enters the body. Foods like bread and cakes have been in our diets for centuries but the majority that are manufactured, like sweets, chocolate, snacks and ice cream, have only been available more recently. The problem with sugar is that it leads to an addiction that is both habitual and social.

Regular annual reports of the British diet over the last thirty years show that sugar consumption has risen from around 14.5kg (32lb) a year per person in 1986, to around 68kg (150lb) per year currently. These figures only include foods eaten within the home and not the sugar in fast food eaten on the go or in restaurants, snacks or school meals. When this is taken into consideration, the total yearly average sugar consumption is more like 82kg (180lb) of sugar per year. If we were to create a brand-new food additive and discovered that it was only a fraction as harmful as sugar, that substance would be quickly banned. As a health educator, I decided that if eating sugar at our current levels is really this dangerous, then everybody should be told about it.

About this book

Recognising the link between food, behaviour and ill health is a huge step. However, it is not a simple case of just cutting out all sugar in the foods you and your children eat. This is especially so because children don't see anything wrong in having a can of Coke and a bag of crisps as they walk to school with their friends who are all doing the same – there are no health warnings on products that contain sugar. This also means that children are not committed to replacing sweet foods with nutritious alternatives.

When researching the foods children were eating, I found that many did not eat breakfast and most ate meals and snacks throughout the day composed of refined carbohydrates with a high sugar content. A sweet tooth begins in babyhood, so children often automatically request or seek out high-sugar drinks rather than opting for water when they are thirsty. Avoidance is the only way to stop the body being addicted to sugar: smoking in moderation doesn't allow the body to quit a nicotine addiction and the same goes for eating sugar. The only difference is that food is essential for life despite the fact it contains sugar, while nicotine from cigarettes is not a necessity.

We are currently bombarded with information about eating a healthy diet and what we should be feeding ourselves and our children. By reading this book, you will discover why sugar has harmful effects on the body. It is important to know what you and your children are eating and how to reduce the amount of sugar consumed to prevent these problems. I know how hard it is to make the best decision you can about a healthy diet and how this relies on many factors such as knowledge, availability and cost. I will discuss the health issues linked to a high-sugar diet in detail but this subject can be emotive. It's not my intention to cast blame in the information provided as – excuse the pun – I cannot sugar-coat the truth. Instead, I will show you how to reduce your child's sugar intake and help you make healthier food choices so that you can be proactive in preventing health problems.

Advertisements emphasise that a product is fine to eat as 'part of a balanced diet'. This statement disguises the fact that eating sugar regularly is a risk factor for obesity, hypertension (high blood pressure), Type 2 diabetes, fatty liver disease and behavioural problems like hyperactivity. If a child or adult is having a can of Coke and a bag of crisps for breakfast or lunch, that is not a balanced diet. If I manage to persuade you to adopt a lifestyle change avoiding all or nearly all added sugar, writing this book will have been completely worthwhile and you will reap the benefits by reading it. 'Giving up sugar' suggests that you will be deprived in some way, like going on a strict diet. *How to Reduce Your Child's Sugar Intake* does not rely on willpower – it's not a temporary fix, it is a lifestyle change. A sugar addiction cannot be tackled with willpower or going without. I will show how this can be achieved.

SUGAR ISN'T LOVE

The Trouble with Sugar

For a long time, the emphasis has been on fat as the worst thing we eat, but as the epidemic of Type 2 diabetes, obesity and heart disease escalates, sugar has now taken that mantle. While we are now far more cautious about the type and amount of fat we consume, added sugars attract less attention. The irony is that lower-fat foods tend to contain more sugar to make their taste appealing.

Confirming a definite link between eating sugar and the development of health problems like Type 2 diabetes has been difficult because a number of factors are involved. It was previously only possible to suggest that a high-sugar diet significantly increases the risk of developing Type 2 diabetes, or any other health condition. Added to this, research focused on studies using high levels of sugar to accelerate the disease process in rats that might take years to occur in a human being, making the timescale of effects associated with sugar difficult to identify. Despite this, growing evidence has recently shown direct links between sugar and disease,[1] so it is now possible to say, without doubt, that sugar is a poisonous, toxic substance that should be eliminated from the diet as far as possible.

Sources of dietary sugars

Carbohydrates provide energy and, along with protein, allow for the formation of muscle. The body needs a constant supply of energy and the raw materials for growth and repair – especially for children – from food and drink. Our bodies break down carbohydrates into the simple sugars glucose, fructose and galactose. All other forms of sugar, such as sucrose, lactose and maltose, are combinations of these three simple sugars.

The building blocks of all carbohydrates are sugars. Sugars are classified according to how many saccharides – sugar units – are contained in one molecule. Glucose, fructose and galactose are single unit sugars, also called monosaccharides. Sugars with double units are called disaccharides, such as sucrose (table sugar) made up of one molecule of glucose and one molecule of fructose, or lactose (milk sugar) which is made up of a molecule of galactose and a molecule of glucose.

FACT: _____

Naturally occurring sugars such as fructose in fruit and lactose in milk are not healthier than the sugars added to food and drink by manufacturers.

FACT: _____

In the UK, baby milk and 'growing-up milk' for toddlers contain fructose – fruit sugar – as a sweetener because formulas containing sucrose – sugar – are banned. This is not the case in other countries.

We have evolved to tolerate milk sugar – lactose from cow's milk – in our diet. As we grow older, lactose can upset the digestive system and cause problems such as diarrhoea because our bodies fail to produce an enzyme that allows lactose to be broken down into galactose and glucose. As with fructose, lactose may be tolerated in small amounts but if the enzyme required to break lactose down is not produced by the body, the individual develops lactose intolerance. While soya milk is marketed as an alternative for those with lactose intolerance, it contains white cane sugar rather than lactose to make it palatable.

FACT: _____

Cow's milk with added galactose and glucose instead of the single-sugar lactose is now available for people with lactose intolerance.

Why excessive sugar is bad for you

A great deal of research has examined the effects on health of including bread, meat, vegetables, eggs and breakfast cereals in our diet, but very few studies have looked solely at the effects of eating foods containing sugar. This is despite the fact that sugar constitutes, on average, about 13.5 per cent of a four- to ten-year-old's diet and this is a larger proportion than any other single food. The meat and dairy industries have carried out extensive and costly nutritional research to support the health effects of their products, even though these foods form a much smaller part of the Western diet when compared with sugar.

FACT:

Worldwide sugar consumption has tripled over the past fifty years.

Lisa says, 'I first began to look more carefully at fruit sugars after our dentist said these could cause tooth decay. My five-year-old daughter loves eating dried fruit and drinking fruit juice because of the sweet taste, but I've now changed that to fresh fruit only and water or milk to drink. The dentist has said that the difference in my daughter's teeth is already noticeable, so I know I'm doing the right thing.'

Because we are told to eat five portions of fruit and vegetables per day – and in some countries, it's eight portions – we have regularly included dried fruits and fruit juices into our diet to meet this total in the belief we are making a healthy choice. However, the guidelines are not clear. Five-a-day is the minimum amount recommended, and if you're trying to reduce sugar in the family diet, that should be two pieces of fruit per day and three portions of vegetables for adults and one portion of fruit per day and four portions of vegetables for children because of the fructose present in fruit. There are also varying levels of sugar present in vegetables, especially sweetcorn, sweet potatoes, carrots, beetroot and sugar snap peas, but this is considerably less than the fructose contained in fruit. Dried fruits are not good food choices as they contain concentrated fruit sugar – 75 per cent fructose, while fruit juices contain the equivalent sugar content of a can of non-diet fizzy drink.

FACT: _____

In terms of daily calorie intake, sugar makes up around 13.5 per cent of daily calories for a four- to ten-year-old, and 14.1 per cent for eleven- to eighteen-year-olds. The NHS recommendation is to limit the daily calories contributed by sugar to no more than 5 per cent.

According to a UK National Diet and Nutrition survey in 2018,[2] children are consuming huge amounts of sugar in their diets – typically the equivalent of 4,800 cubes of sugar every year or thirteen cubes per day, which is more than twice the recommended amount for a child aged four to ten. The main sources of sugars forming the diets of children are shown below:

Source of dietary sugar	Percentage
Non-diet soft drinks, juice drinks, energy drinks, colas and other fizzy drinks	10
Buns, cakes, pasties and fruit pies	10
Table sugar, preserves and sweet spreads	9
Biscuits	9
Breakfast cereals	8
Chocolate/confectionery	7
Yoghurt, fromage frais and other dairy desserts	6
Ice cream	5
Puddings	4

FACT: _____

It's never too late to start reducing the amount of sugar in your child's diet. Every 4g of sugar found in a product is equivalent to one teaspoon.

A 2018 study[3] examined 2,019 adults who had developed Type 2 diabetes in association with drinking one can of sugar-sweetened fizzy drink per day versus one diet version of the fizzy drink per day. Results showed a 95 per cent association between consuming the sugary drink and the onset of Type 2 diabetes. Type 2 diabetes develops when the body is unable to control blood glucose levels effectively so that more and more insulin is produced to bring glucose levels under control; this in turn leads to weight gain because insulin encourages fat to be stored. When there is fat present around body cells, insulin cannot work properly. The researchers suggested that the development of Type 2 diabetes in those consuming diet drinks was due to their having an increased body mass index – these participants were overweight. It is known that it can take up to twelve years before Type 2 diabetes is diagnosed because symptoms are mild, so over time these individuals may have developed Type 2 diabetes anyway. Those participants consuming one sugary drink per day had added to their weight gain in this way.

FACT: _____

One 330ml can of Coke contains 140 calories from sugar.

The very many effects of sugar in the diet include the development of an enlarged and fatty liver, enlarged kidneys and a reduced lifespan. Sugar, specifically fructose eaten daily, also has the effect of increasing the amount of cholesterol and other fats, known as triglycerides, in the bloodstream. Adults cannot deal with more than 10g of fructose per day and the effect is even more significant for children. The effect sugar has on the body can be seen in many ways in terms of increasing the risk of developing or worsening certain health conditions, but if we concentrate initially on the effects of sugar as it travels through the digestive system, we can see the unique way that sugar behaves.

Once something sweet is eaten, acids and bacteria increase within the mouth to attack tooth enamel before the sugar travels into the stomach to irritate the stomach lining as it is digested. We know that sugar stimulates the adrenal glands which in turn increase the amount of stomach acid produced. Sugar eaten on an empty stomach acts as an irritant: studies show that swallowing a solution containing four lumps of sugar on an empty stomach causes the stomach lining to become red and inflamed. In the same way, heartburn or reflux – when stomach acid rises up the oesophagus and burns – can be caused by a high sugar diet, where more stomach acid is produced. If sugary foods are eaten too often, the result can be a duodenal ulcer caused by increased hydrochloric acid levels in the stomach.

Once absorbed into the digestive system, sugar becomes blood glucose and this travels to every part of the body. If the body cannot manage glucose levels by producing insulin to normalise blood glucose, this state is known as pre-diabetes. A higher blood glucose level means the blood has increased acidity, disrupting the metabolism because it cannot work properly. In the intestines, a high-sugar diet can decrease the number of good bacteria in the gut. This imbalance leads to increased sugar cravings which can cause further intestinal disruption. A diet that is high in refined sugars, particularly high-fructose corn syrup, has been linked to increased inflammation throughout the body.

Paul says, 'I had been feeling frequently tired but thought it was due to work pressures. A routine health check showed elevated blood glucose levels. This test was repeated by my doctor and still showed a higher than normal level of glucose. I told the doctor I'd been craving sweet things and he said this was because my body was no longer able to process glucose in the same way and I craved sweet things to provide my body cells with energy. A diagnosis of pre-diabetes was made and I was advised to eat a low-sugar diet. The next two blood tests showed normal levels of glucose and I no longer feel tired.'

Effects of sugar on the body

- Sugar is as addictive as nicotine, alcohol, morphine and heroin, and has similar effects on the brain.

- Sugar causes the kidneys, liver and adrenal glands on top of the kidneys to become enlarged (hyperplasia), causing swelling and increasing cell growth (hypertrophy).

- Sugar increases blood insulin levels, as well as adrenal cortical hormone and oestrogen levels. This occurs when the blood glucose and fructose concentration is high following the digestion of sucrose – cane or beet sugar.

- Raised glucose levels and an insulin imbalance is a risk factor for many health conditions, such as Type 2 diabetes, cancer and polycystic ovary syndrome (PCOS). An increased level of one hormone in the body has an adverse impact on the body's metabolism, leading to an increase or decrease in other hormones.

- Sugar increases the release of the hormone ghrelin, which stimulates appetite, hunger and promotes fat storage. Sugar also decreases the normal action of the hormone leptin, which promotes the burning of fat for energy when carbohydrates are in short supply. The action of sugar on ghrelin and leptin leads to weight gain.

- Sugar causes a change in cell enzymes so that over a number of years, body cells are less able to function in the normal way. This is true of increased blood glucose levels in diabetes, where cells are unable to use glucose as fuel if too much glucose is present in the blood and white blood cells are less able to fight infection.

FACT: _____

When large amounts of sugar are consumed, this cannot be absorbed correctly and some of this undigested sucrose enters the bloodstream.

How much is too much?

While there is no consistent health guideline for total daily sugars, 90g is suggested on food labelling in Britain and across the EU. This equates to around twenty-two teaspoons of sugar per day. In the US, the 'average' adult intake is suggested as 77g of sugar per day. One white sugar cube weighs 4g and contains three-quarters of a teaspoon of sugar and sixteen calories. According to the NHS, adults should eat no more than 30g of sugars a day – roughly equivalent to seven sugar cubes or 112 calories from sugar. Children aged seven to ten should eat no more than 24g of sugars a day – six sugar cubes or 96 calories from sugar. Children aged four to six should eat no more than 19g of sugars a day – five sugar cubes or 80 calories from sugar.

FACT: _____

Added sugar from processed foods has no place in a healthy diet, especially if you or your child has a weight problem or diabetes.

As you can see, with differing guidelines between the manufacturing industry and the NHS on how much sugar we should or should not be eating, the subject becomes very confusing.

Added sugars – by food manufacturers, the cook or consumer – are among the most controversial and hotly debated topics in nutrition, but there is little doubt that added sugar is the single worst ingredient in the modern diet. As we have already seen, sugar has no nutritional value and it disrupts the metabolism, leading to the development of serious health problems like obesity, Type 2 diabetes and heart disease. Sugary foods have the same effect on the brain as heroin or morphine although a sugar addiction is far easier to overcome. It is important to decide how strict you are going to be on sugar consumption as it's impossible to avoid all types of sugar unless you grow all your own food and make your own meals from scratch without adding any types of sugar.

FACT: _____

It is very important to recognise the difference between the added sugars in manufactured foods and sugars that occur naturally in foods like fruits and vegetables that also contain fibre and valuable nutrients.

It is difficult to measure the level of sugars an adult or child consumes because this relies on self-reporting and keeping meticulous food diaries, so very little research is available in this respect, although we do know that daily sugar consumption varies greatly from person to person. You may be confused by the different descriptions of sugar in food, such as 'total sugars', 'added sugars' and 'free sugars', so I will now explain the difference.

Total sugars describe all naturally occurring sugars present in the product from sources such as fruit and milk. Sucrose is naturally present in foods such as fruits.

Added sugars describe the sugars added to foods by the manufacturer, cook or consumer, such as sucrose, fructose, glucose, high-fructose syrup or concentrated fruit juice, some of which are naturally present in food. Added sugars are extracted or produced from naturally occurring sources such as glucose or fructose from fruits, vegetables, honey or milk. This means that whether the sugar consumed is from a biscuit or a piece of fruit, the component sugars it contains remain structurally the same so sugar is sugar, from whatever source. Added sugars may be part of foods with a low nutritional value or as an intact source, such as a piece of fruit, where they are accompanied by other nutrients and fibre.

Free sugars describe added sugars plus sugars that are naturally present in honey, syrup and fruit juices.

Simplifying all sources of sugar eaten as a whole is also difficult because research studies break down each source of sugar separately to provide complex data, including other factors such as ethnicity or health conditions that are already present in the participants. I have found the best source of information about daily sugar intake by age and gender to be the insightful book *Pure, White and Deadly*,[4] first published in 1972 by physiologist and nutritionist Professor John Yudkin and reprinted in 2012. The daily intake for sugars stated below is now far greater more than forty years on, but the overall outcome is still the same: teenage boys tend to consume more daily sugars than teenage girls and people in their sixties eat around one-third less sugar than those in their twenties.

Daily sugar intake in grams by age and gender (1972)		
Age	**Male**	**Female**
15–19	156	96
20–29	112	101
30–39	126	100
40–49	96	83
50–59	90	83
60–69	92	63

FACT: _____

Added sugar is the main ingredient in confectionery and in many processed foods like soft drinks and bakery items. The most common added sugars are what we know as table sugar (sucrose)

and high-fructose corn syrup (HFCS). HFCS is a sweetener derived from corn syrup, which is processed from corn. It is primarily used in the United States to sweeten processed foods and soft drinks.

It is estimated that depending on the amount eaten, confectionery currently constitutes 7 per cent of daily sugars for children, although this may be far more for some. In addition to this daily average for confectionery, sugar intake rises with the amount of sweet cereal, fizzy drinks, cakes, biscuits, ice cream and other desserts consumed by young people. The estimate for the average amount of sugar eaten by a thirteen-year-old constitutes 850–1,000 calories of their 3,000-calorie daily total eaten as sugar. Some children eat far more than this average, meaning that as much as half of the recommended daily calorie allowance for children is coming from sugar. A 2018 study has shown that during the school summer holidays, children will, on average, eat five times more sugar.[5]

FACT: _____

People in Britain eat more chocolate per head than any other nation. The equivalent of 540 Kit Kat bars are eaten every second in the UK.

When words like 'average' are used to describe sugar consumption, this is again difficult to quantify. The word 'average' is used interchangeably with the word 'moderate' to mean the amount someone might eat or drink in a given time period, or how much a person might exercise. This causes confusion when we are told to do things in moderation in order to protect our health, such as eating less sugar. It was once considered that eating an ounce (28.3g) of sugar every day was moderate, but now we eat around five ounces, equivalent to 141.5g a day, so the boundaries have changed regarding how much is acceptable.

KEY MESSAGES IN THIS CHAPTER

- There is no need for added sugars in a healthy diet.

- Consuming a diet high in sugar that's added to processed foods is much worse than eating the sugar contained in fruit (fructose) as fruit is eaten in smaller quantities.

- High sugar intake is associated with various lifestyle diseases including obesity, Type 2 diabetes and heart disease.

- Eating a diet high in processed foods makes it difficult to reduce or avoid added sugar.

- The NHS advises that adults should eat no more than 30g – just over an ounce – of free sugars a day, roughly equivalent to seven sugar cubes or 112 calories from sugar that is added to foods. Free sugars are the types of sugar that can cause health problems for children and adults. Children aged seven to ten should eat no more than 24g of free sugars a day, equivalent to six sugar cubes or 96 calories from sugar. Children aged four to six should eat no more than 19g of free sugars a day – five sugar cubes or 80 calories from sugar.

- Sugar intake can be significantly reduced by cutting out soft drinks, confectionery, fruit juice and bakery items.

Starches and Sugars

The word 'sugar' has a double meaning as it is used to refer to the amount of glucose entering the blood after a meal (blood sugar) as well as the sugar we use in our homes or what is added to food and drink by manufacturers. Blood sugar is really the amount of glucose in the blood while sugars such as glucose and sucrose are carbohydrates. Some carbohydrates can be digested in the gut and others cannot. Those that cannot be digested form the dietary fibre that passes through the body virtually unchanged. Digested carbohydrates mostly consist of sugars and starch.

Refined carbohydrates like white flour have the most nutritious part of the grain – that provides fibre – removed, so refined carbohydrates are broken down very quickly by the body and blood glucose increases rapidly. White flour is used to make white bread, rolls, baguettes, pancakes, tortillas, waffles, muffins, crumpets, bagels, noodles and white pasta. Complex carbohydrates such as whole grains, beans, potatoes and roots take much longer to raise blood glucose because the body has to work hard to obtain energy from these foods.

FACT: _____

Starch is the stored energy found in plants and is made up of many units of glucose. When starch is broken down in the body it becomes maltose and eventually glucose.

Sources of starch

Bread, pasta, potatoes, rice, breakfast cereals, oats and other grains such as rye and barley are starchy foods. Although these foods are often referred to as 'carbs', this is not strictly the case as carbohydrates include both starch and sugars, as well as fibre. Starchy foods provide us with energy because they are broken down into glucose for brain and muscle fuel. Starchy foods are also nutrient-rich, providing a source of B vitamins, iron and calcium; 50 per cent of our daily calories should come from these carbohydrates. Starchy foods such as brown rice and wholewheat pasta are also a good source of fibre necessary for a healthy digestive system to lower the risk of heart disease, stroke, Type 2 diabetes and bowel cancer.

TIP:
Always choose cereals that have a better fibre content than sugary cereals as the fibre will mean blood glucose levels rise more evenly after eating.

Choose starchy carbohydrates that provide more fibre such as wholegrain or wholemeal bread, wholewheat pasta, brown rice, and leave the skin on potatoes. The recommended level of daily fibre is 30g for adults. Children of one to three years should have 19g of fibre per day, while children of four to eight years should have 25g of fibre per day. Boys aged nine to thirteen years should have 31g of fibre per day, while girls of the same age should have 26 grams per day. Despite the fact that starchy carbohydrates should make up around a third of our daily diet, in the UK starchy carbohydrates only make up one-fifth of the food we consume.

FACT:
Refined carbohydrates satisfy the appetite because they contain starch or sugar in some form. They are found in manufactured foods such as bread, cakes and biscuits.

Different types of sugar

Glucose is a simple sugar that provides our main source of energy. Glucose is found in most foods with the exception of meat, although meat is broken down by our bodies to provide some glucose for energy.

Our bodies use glucose for energy to power the brain, muscles and chemical reactions that control ordinary bodily functions. Glucose is a type of sugar that comes from the breakdown of carbohydrates (starches) like bread, potatoes and pasta. Sugar is a simple carbohydrate that breaks down into glucose in the body. Eating either glucose or sugar – or the carbohydrates that turn into them as they are processed by the body – increase blood glucose levels. Glucose is also found with other sugars in certain fruits and vegetables.

Fructose is found in ripe fruits and combines with glucose to give a sweet taste. Fructose is also found in honey (40 per cent fructose), maple syrup (40 per cent fructose) and agave syrup (90 per cent fructose). Fructose with some glucose and sucrose is found in fruit.

Lactose is a sugar found in milk that is composed of galactose and glucose subunits. Lactose makes up around 2–8 per cent of milk by weight.

Maltose is produced during the digestion of starch which is broken down into glucose. Many of our foods are converted into glucose where it is metabolised by the body to provide energy.

Galactose is found in dairy products such as yoghurt where lactose joins with glucose.

Sucrose – refined cane or beet table sugar – is a combination of glucose and fructose. Caster sugar is also sucrose that has finer grains. Other forms of sucrose are brown sugar and raw sugar. Sucrose is the chemical name for sugar.

FACT: _____

As fruit ripens the glucose it contains is converted into fructose – fruit sugar.

Primary sources of glucose in the diet are bread, potatoes and pasta that are broken down by the body to use as fuel for energy. Sugar is a secondary source of energy that has to be broken down into glucose. Glucose is always circulating in the bloodstream and is known as 'blood glucose'. Eating sugar or starch means the level of blood glucose is raised by the glucose in food and drink. To lower blood glucose back to normal levels, insulin is released by the pancreas and the glucose is converted into a substance called glycogen that is stored in the liver and muscles to be used when glucose levels are too low. The human body only has 350g of stored glycogen.

Glycaemic index

Glycaemic index (GI) is a value assigned to carbohydrate foods based on how quickly or slowly they are digested to increase blood glucose levels. The glycaemic index was created to rank the foods that cause spikes in blood glucose. The food is typically ranked out of 100, with 100 being the greatest increase in blood glucose. Carbohydrates with a low GI – usually 55 or less – are digested and absorbed more slowly, therefore blood glucose levels do not shoot up. Chocolate, lactose and fructose have low GI values, while sucrose has an intermediate GI value. Diets containing more low GI foods are associated with a reduced risk of developing metabolic diseases like Type 2 diabetes. Foods with a high GI – greater than 70 – containing glucose and maltose are digested quickly and cause blood glucose and insulin levels to increase rapidly. This is not advisable for children or people with diabetes and can cause health problems like heart disease and obesity. The blood glucose response is influenced by the combination of the GI value of different foods and the total amount of consumed carbohydrate.

FACT: _____

High blood insulin levels increase hunger and encourage the body to store fat.

Eating a low GI food along with fat, protein or other carbohydrates reduces the GI value further, so eating a cheese sandwich means the GI value of the wholegrain bread is changed by the consumption of the protein and fat in cheese. It can also be the case that the method of food preparation can change the GI value of certain foods – for example, whether it is fried in oil or grilled with no oil. The ripeness and age of fruits and vegetables also alters their GI value – unripe fruits tend to have a lower GI than ripe fruit containing more fructose and, similarly, older potatoes contain more starch than new potatoes. It is important to include fruit in the daily diet for you and your child but it's best to choose fruit that ranks low on the glycaemic index. Here are some fruits that have a low GI value:

- Berries – 65g serving

- Figs – a serving of four fresh or dried

- Cherries – 103g fresh sour cherries with stones

- Pears – one medium 178g

- Apples – one medium 138g

- Peaches – one medium 147g

- Grapefruit – one, without skin, 230g

Adi says, 'I was looking to lose weight and did some research into the glycaemic index of foods. While it can be difficult to calculate the exact value of what I feed the family because how the food is prepared can make a difference, it is really worth looking into. We have been eating low GI foods for six months now and my husband and two teenage boys agree they feel so much better without the spikes in blood glucose levels they had before we made this change. We are a happier and healthier family.'

Highly processed carbohydrate-rich foods have the highest glycaemic index value, such as grains with the fibre content removed – white bread, white pasta and white rice, for example. Fibre helps to slow down digestion so it reduces the glycaemic index. Because various factors can affect the glycaemic index of a food, it can be difficult to adopt a low GI diet and be sure a food won't raise blood glucose levels quickly. These complexities mean that the GI diet is not taught by diabetes clinics to people with diabetes to help manage the condition.

FACT:

Highly processed foods like white bread, doughnuts, bagels and many processed breakfast cereals lack fibre, so they have a high glycaemic index.

The following list will help you make food choices with a lower glycaemic index to prevent a sharp increase in blood glucose levels:

- Use brown basmati rice instead of white rice or white pasta, and wholewheat or gluten-free noodles instead of those made with white flour. You could substitute quinoa, which is gluten-free, high in protein and contains all nine essential amino acids. Quinoa is also high in fibre, magnesium, B vitamins, iron, potassium, calcium, phosphorus, vitamin E and various beneficial antioxidants.

- Eat wholemeal roti – flatbreads made from stoneground, wholemeal flour, and include lentils and pulses in your meals.

- Use new potatoes instead of old potatoes.

- Instead of white bread, choose granary, pumpernickel or rye bread.

- Substitute wholewheat noodles or wholewheat pasta for frozen chips. Rinse pasta or noodles in boiling water once cooked to reduce the starch content further.

- Try porridge or wholegrain breakfast cereals instead of cornflakes or puffed rice cereal.

What's different about fructose?

One particular form of sugar – fructose, or fruit sugar – does not behave in the same way as other carbohydrates. When we eat fruit sugar, around 1 per cent of undigested fructose is directly converted to plasma triglyceride – blood fats. The liver converts one-third to one-half of fructose into glucose, and about a quarter of fructose becomes lactic acid which allows glucose to be used as energy. Any remaining fructose is converted into glycogen – stored energy. Our growing consumption of sugar has radically increased our fructose intake, used by manufacturers because it is sweeter than sugar. The major source of fructose in the diet comes from sugar, sweetened drinks via fructose-containing sugars, sucrose and high-fructose corn syrup. Regular consumption of sugary drinks sweetened with fructose can lead to weight gain because the calories they contain are not filling and people tend to consume the calories from these drinks as well as their normal meals. It is known that fructose affects the body in several different ways:

- Fructose disrupts the body's metabolism of copper, affecting the production of collagen and elastin in muscles and organs, and iodine metabolism, necessary for a healthy thyroid gland.

- Fructose has been recognised as causing persistently high blood glucose levels. This is equivalent to untreated diabetes and over time high blood glucose levels can cause damage to every cell, especially the eyes, nerves, kidneys, blood vessels and heart.

- Fructose has a negative effect on the body, increasing blood pressure and levels of blood fats (triglycerides), hormone secretion, depression and the accumulation of body fat around the central organs.

- A high level of blood fats may lead to fatty liver disease and insulin resistance, a key risk factor for developing Type 2 diabetes and cardiovascular disease. Overconsumption of fructose can also lead to too much uric acid in the blood, which is associated with gout, a painful inflammatory arthritis.

- High consumption of fructose can increase cortisol levels. Cortisol is the stress hormone that increases blood pressure and suppresses the immune system when we feel pressured or tense, causing anxiety.

Dionne says, 'You think you're being healthy, eating lots of fruit and giving your kids fruit juice instead of Coke to drink. Then I saw a TV programme about the dangers of eating too much fruit. Consumers don't realise that it's fresh fruit that's important as it contains fibre to offset the fructose, so it is beneficial in the diet. What you should not buy is the processed fruit treats and drinks that have little or no fibre and a massive dose of fruit sugar.'

Following Easter, Halloween and Christmas – times of increased sugar consumption – rates of cold and flu rapidly increase in children due to excess dietary sugars reducing the white blood cell count, making children more vulnerable to infection. Fructose has been shown to raise cortisol levels without being triggered by stress every time sugar is consumed, and this cortisol response can happen multiple times a day in response to fructose. In terms of weight gain, limiting intake of sugar-sweetened beverages or added sugars will have a measurable impact on weight control and prevention of lifestyle diseases.

Consuming one non-diet fizzy drink each day has been linked to:

- The risk of developing Type 2 diabetes being increased by 25 per cent

- The risk of heart attack or developing fatal heart disease increasing by 35 per cent

- The risk of having a stroke increasing by 16 per cent.

It is difficult to know exactly how much fructose is contained in fruit because it doesn't come with a label. Be aware that children should only have one piece of fruit a day, while the limit for adults is two pieces. Health advice now tells us that we should be eating seven a day, but that target is the ideal for adults meaning two fruits and five vegetables, not eating fruit or vegetables that amount to seven portions. While vegetables such as beetroot, sweetcorn and carrots contain more fructose than other vegetables, this is far less than the content in fruit so even the sweetest vegetables are equivalent to fruits with a low fructose content.

Some advertisements say that fruit and vegetable juices are 'one of your five-a-day' but if the fibre is removed these concentrated juice products should be avoided. Eating fresh fruit with nuts and seeds provides the best solution to adding fibre and reducing any damage from excess fructose.

Children love eating berries. Adding frozen berries to a packed lunch is an easy way to include a portion of fruit in your child's diet. You can also make sandwiches in advance for the whole week and freeze them for children's lunches if you are pushed for time in the mornings.

The difference between primary carbohydrates and added sugars

Natural sugars that are contained in foods like vegetables and milk are not the kind that can cause health problems: these natural sugars are included in the total sugars found in the foods we buy and there is no need to cut these out of either your or your child's diet. The type of sugars in the diet that can lead to health problems for adults and children if eaten to excess are known as *free sugars*. Free sugars are classed in two groups:

- Sugars added to food and drinks such as breakfast cereals, flavoured yoghurts, fizzy drinks, biscuits and chocolate. Additional sugar may be added at home, for example to cereals, or added during the manufacturing process to enhance the flavour of the food.

- Sugars occurring in honey and products such as golden or maple syrup, unsweetened fruit or vegetable juices and smoothies. Although these sugars appear naturally in the ingredients, they are concentrated in these products so they are classed as free sugars.

Manufacturers and supermarkets have been urged to simplify the amount of dietary sugars in their products by using traffic-light colours so consumers can see this information at a glance. The traffic-light system includes green sugars: sugars that occur naturally as carbohydrates in foods; amber sugars: natural sugars that are concentrated in fruit juices and smoothies, honey and syrups; and red sugars: additional sugars added during the cooking or manufacturing process.

Food labelling – the traffic-light system explained

Food labelling gives you information about the number of calories – energy, protein, fat, saturated fat, sugar and salt – that you and your family are eating. This nutritional information is given per 100g of food and some manufacturers also provide values per portion. You can use this information to help you chose low-sugar foods, as well as foods that are lower in fat and salt. Ingredients are listed by weight so you can see how much sugar the product has.

What is classified as a high level of fat, sugar or salt?

The nutritional information on food about the amount of fat, sugar and salt it contains is given as a guideline.

Total fat: A food is high in fat if it contains more than 17.5g of fat per 100g. It is low in fat if it contains 3g of fat or less per 100g.

Saturated fat: A food is high in saturated – unhealthy – fat if it contains more than 5g of saturated fat per 100g. It is low in saturated fat if it contains 1.5g of saturated fat or less per 100g.

Sugars: A food is high in sugars if it contains more than 22.5g of total sugars per 100g. It is low in sugars if it contains 5g of total sugars or less per 100g.

Salt or sodium: A food is high in salt if it contains more than 1.5g of salt per 100g or 0.6g of sodium. A food is low in salt if it contains 0.3g of salt or less per 100g or 0.1g of sodium.

Colour-coded information is now given by food manufacturers and supermarkets on the front of packaging so you can see at a glance how much energy, fat, saturated fat, sugars and salt is in the food. Food labelling also provides information about 'reference intakes' which are the recommended daily amounts of, for example, sugars or saturated fat.

TIP: _____

Always check what the manufacturer recommends as a portion size – a family bag of crisps containing 'eight portions' may be shared between two people, for example, so nutritional values for the amount eaten need to be calculated for half the bag each instead.

The traffic-light system of labelling food with a section of red, amber and green colours on the front of the packaging allows you to see instantly whether the food is high, medium or low in calories, saturated fat, sugars or salt. Red indicates high so these foods should be consumed with caution or not bought at all; amber means medium, so the food is neither high nor low and can be eaten as and when you like; green indicates low, so it is a healthy choice.

If you are comparing similar products that don't have traffic-light coding, look at the ingredients list and see where sugars are listed. If any of the sugars are first, second or third on the list, then it's a high-sugar food. The same goes for fats. If foods are marked 'low sugar' it means they contain no more than 5 per cent sugar per 100g/100ml of food or drink. Foods marked 'high sugar' have 15g of sugar or more per 100g/100ml.

KEY MESSAGES IN THIS CHAPTER

- Refined carbohydrates such as white flour provide little fibre, and are broken down very quickly and raise blood glucose rapidly. White flour is used to make white bread, rolls, baguettes, pancakes, tortillas, waffles, muffins, crumpets, bagels, noodles and white pasta.

- Complex carbohydrates such as whole grains, beans, potatoes and roots take much longer to raise blood glucose because the body has to work hard to obtain energy from these foods. Bread, pasta, potatoes, rice, breakfast cereals, oats and other grains such as rye and barley are starchy foods. Starchy foods provide us with energy because they are broken down into glucose for brain and muscle fuel.

- The recommended level of daily fibre is 30g for adults. Children of one to three years should have 19g of fibre per day, while children of four to eight years should have 25g of fibre per day. Boys aged nine to thirteen years should have 31g of fibre per day, while girls of the same age should have 26g per day.

- Regular consumption of sugary drinks sweetened with fructose can lead to weight gain because the calories they contain are not filling.

- Free sugars in the diet can lead to health problems if eaten to excess. Free sugars are sugars added to food and drinks such as breakfast cereals, flavoured yoghurts, fizzy drinks, biscuits and chocolate. Additional sugar may be added at home, for example, to cereals, or during the manufacturing process. Free sugars also occur in honey, golden or maple syrup, unsweetened fruit or vegetable juices and smoothies. Although these sugars appear naturally in the ingredients, they are concentrated in these products.

- Traffic-light labelling on foods: red indicates high so these foods should be consumed with caution or not bought at all; amber means medium, so the food is neither high nor low and can be eaten as and when you like; green indicates low, so it is a healthy choice.

Government Action on Sugar

Many countries, including the UK, have introduced a sugar tax. This is intended to reduce sugar consumption either directly or indirectly. A direct sugar tax increases the cost of all fizzy drinks so that consumers do not buy them at all, or they buy less of the product. An indirect sugar tax is applied by manufacturers and retailers who change their products, reduce portion sizes or change product lines by introducing healthier alternatives. Currently, there's no global definition of how much sugar constitutes a high-sugar drink but regulations exist for the level of sugar where taxes are introduced. The UK introduced taxes on soft drinks that contain 8g of sugar per 100ml.[1] This is not the same in South Africa, where half of the UK amount of sugar – 4g – is taxed in soft drinks. Mexico introduced its tax on sugary drinks in January 2014 because more than 70 per cent of Mexicans were overweight or obese,[2] increasing the cost of sugary drinks for the consumer and introducing an 8 per cent tax on foods containing high levels of sugar, salt and fat. Many other countries have since followed this example.

The UK Government introduced the Soft Drinks Industry Levy (SDIL) in April 2018 as part of the Government's childhood obesity strategy. This tax puts a charge of 24p on drinks containing 8g of sugar per 100ml and 18p a litre on those with 5–8g of sugar per 100ml, directly payable by manufacturers to HM Revenue and Customs (HMRC). The tax attempts to control sugar consumption via soft drinks, especially by children, with the aim of persuading manufacturers to reduce the amount of sugar the drinks contain so they don't have to pay this levy, therefore providing the consumer with a healthier version of the product. This levy is similar to the taxes on alcohol and tobacco; as we have already seen, sugar is an addictive substance in the same way as alcohol and nicotine. The 'sugar' tax aims to address a market crisis brought about by products that cause health concerns where the cost to health has not been included in the product price.

What the Government says

Because the consumption of sugar is not currently regarded as a danger to public health, there are no restrictions on purchasing sugar or foods containing sugar. In 2017, Public Health England (PHE) called for a 20 per cent reduction in the sugar content of food produce by 2020, with a suggested 5 per cent target for the first year. However, a PHE report released in May 2018 found that many food manufacturers and supermarkets have not managed to reach this target. The Government had also promised a ban on the sale of energy drinks to under-sixteens, but this has not happened to date.

Since the introduction of the SDIL in April 2018, the UK Treasury department has received less revenue than expected from this measure: over 50 per cent of soft drink manufacturers, including Ribena, Lucozade and Fanta, have opted to change the recipe of their drinks to reduce the sugar content rather than pay the charge, so this is better for consumers. The Government now estimates they will receive £240 million from the remaining 50 per cent of manufacturers such as Coke Classic and Original Pepsi that have not acted to reduce sugar in their product since the introduction of the levy. There is no evidence to show that the indirect tax on sugary drinks has made any difference to the amount consumed by the public, even when prices were increased in a direct tax to consumers. Rates of Type 2 diabetes, obesity and heart disease continue to rise and children are still consuming these drinks, laying the foundations for health problems in the future.

FACT: _____

In September 2019, the Chancellor admitted that the Treasury has pocketed taxes raised through the soft drinks sugar levy that were supposed to support children's health.

The consumption of fat was once seen as being at the root of all chronic disease such as Type 2 diabetes, stroke, heart disease, fatty liver disease and some cancers, but there has been a change in thinking so the focus is now on the destructive power of sugar. Public Health England have pushed for change and insisted that adults and children over the age of eleven should have no more than 30g of sugar per day and that sugar should make up no more than 5 per cent of daily calories. Despite this guideline, no amount of sugar in the diet is safe. It should not be assumed that if a government body says it's fine to eat 30g – just over one ounce – of sugar per day then this will protect against the development of future chronic health problems. Reducing the amount of sugar in the diet will help to reduce the risk of health issues, but simply cutting down on sugar does not break the addiction.

FACT: _____

Clearer product labelling is necessary for parents and children to better assess the amount of sugar contained in foods so they can make an informed decision.

What can the Government do to help tackle obesity?

Sugar is everywhere, with easy access to cheap, processed food making it simple for children and adults alike to consume a great number of calories each day from sweets, chocolate or fizzy drinks without realising it. Even savoury foods aren't safe because manufacturers add sugar to these to make them taste good.

In 2015, Public Health England published 'Sugar reduction: the evidence for action' which described the extent of the threat sugar poses to health, especially to the future health of our children. PHE identified a number of factors that make us more likely to eat sweet foods, including:

• Advertising and marketing promotions that influence us to buy

- Availability of sweet/unhealthy foods and drinks to purchase and consume

- A lack of information and education to enable us to make sensible, low-sugar food choices

It has been suggested by experts that the advertising of high-sugar foods merely persuades us which brands to buy – i.e. a particular brand of cola drink or variety of cake or crisps – rather than encouraging parents and children to buy more of these foods. It has also been recommended that parents should choose foods labelled 'no added sugar' for their children. However, even baby foods with no added sugar still contain sugar: what the manufacturers mean is that the product doesn't contain sucrose or glucose. No added sugar foods are sweetened with honey or fruit juice containing fructose. With this type of misleading information from the manufacturers, even if you do read the food labels carefully, it is no wonder that some parents are confused about what to feed their children when they receive mixed messages about healthy diets and with such a wide choice of foods available.

It is now recognised that sugar impacts on health in two ways: firstly, it leads to obesity and many associated chronic diseases such as Type 2 diabetes, heart disease, stroke, liver disease and some cancers. These diseases were responsible for 72 per cent of deaths in 2016, according to the World Health Organisation. Secondly, sugar has an independent toxic effect on the body aside from causing obesity and related health problems. The toxic effects of sugar affect the whole body, causing inflammation of the cells and tissues so they cannot function correctly. It is difficult for change to occur and more needs to be done by the Government to help families make better food choices.

In June 2018, Public Health England stated that 4,800 cubes of sugar would be consumed per child by the end of that year – more than double the recommended amount. The major contributor to this alarming statistic is the sugar found in fizzy drinks, as well as those added to fruit juices, although they do count towards the five-a-day recommendation for a healthy diet. By July 2019 the UK Government reported that the SDIL (sugar tax) had removed the equivalent of 45,000 tonnes of sugar from soft drinks.[3]

Now the Government has imposed a sugar tax on consumers to try to limit the amount of sugar being eaten, consumers may consider diet drinks or turn to other high-sugar foods to satisfy the craving for sweetness. The main priority of imposing a sugar tax is to conduct research into how much sugar is in certain foods like cereals or fizzy drinks in order to come up with alternatives. Many manufacturers have already reduced the amount of sugar in their products but more needs to be done.

Some sugar alternatives are not healthier options and consumers may think diet drinks are better; but they still provide a sweet taste to fool the brain into thinking it's getting sugar, so this is not helping a sugar dependency. The sugar alternative, aspartame, is used to sweeten some diet drinks although it was discovered that aspartame caused cancer in animal studies.[4] Although aspartame is not used for this reason in some countries, the studies suggesting this sweetener could cause cancer involved high amounts fed to rats over a short period of time. This would be far more aspartame than a human would ever consume so it is felt to be safe, with consumption being down to personal choice.

The UK Government's 'Childhood Obesity Plan for Action'

The Childhood Obesity Plan for Action, produced in 2016, outlined the action the Government will take towards its goal of halving childhood obesity levels and reducing the inequalities among children with obesity from the most deprived areas by 2030. While your child may not be overweight, the consumption of a high-sugar diet is known to significantly contribute to excess weight gain and associated health issues.

Evidence shows that slowly changing the amount of sugar, salt and fat in foods, or reducing product size, is a successful way to make products healthier. This is because the changes are universal and do not rely on individual behavioural changes. The Government aims to launch a widespread, structured sugar reduction programme to remove sugar from the products children eat most often. All sectors of the food and drinks industry were challenged to reduce overall sugar content across a range of products that contribute to children's sugar intakes by at least 20 per cent by 2020. This was attempted by lowering sugar levels in products, reducing portion sizes or changing to lower-sugar alternatives.

PHE are running the Childhood Obesity Plan for Action and this will apply to retailers, manufacturers, restaurants, takeaways and cafés, and to all foods and drinks that contribute to children's sugar intakes, including baby and toddler foods. The programme has initially focused on foods that make the largest contributions to children's sugar intakes: breakfast cereals, yoghurts, biscuits, cakes, confectionery, pastries, puddings, ice cream and sweet spreads. Later work will focus on milk-based drinks and foods for babies and young children. PHE has advised the Government on setting sugar targets per 100g of product and calorie caps for specific single-serving products. Progress will be measured via sales of average sugar content per 100g of food and drink versus foods with reduced portion size so that these contain less sugar to assess a move towards lower-sugar alternatives.

A PHE report has described progress as good after the first year (2018), with manufacturers reducing the amount of sugar and calories in their products by 2 per cent. Of the eight key food category targets, there have been reductions in sugar levels in five categories: yoghurts and fromage frais have seen a 6 per cent reduction in sugar and calories, while breakfast cereals and sweet spreads have seen a 5 per cent reduction in sugar only. Ice cream, lollies and sorbets have seen a 2 per cent reduction in sugar and a 7 per cent reduction in calories. Confectionery and puddings have also seen a 1 per cent reduction in sugar, with puddings now containing 4 per cent fewer calories. Some information is unavailable where the product was not sold as a single-serving portion. Overall, this means that:

- There has been an average 11 per cent reduction in sugar and 6 per cent average calories per portion for retailers' own-label brands and manufacturers' private-label products.

- Shoppers are buying more low-sugar fizzy drinks with less than 5g of sugar per 100g.

It's a family affair

Parents are more than familiar with the battle that ensues in a supermarket when a child decides they want sweets or chocolate. Studies have shown that this argument over wanting to eat sugary snacks occurs when the child first realises it has power over the parent and can use this power to get what it wants. This is not to say that parents are a pushover when a child demands sweets: despite parents' best efforts to protect their children's health, research shows that children nonetheless manage to use deception tactics to get the treats that they want. With the increasing pressures of modern life, it is almost inevitable that parents give in to the easiest option when it comes to demands for snacks and unhealthy foods.

When parents are asked why their children eat sweet foods and drinks, apart from the obvious answer that they like the taste, several themes emerge:

- Sweet foods are readily available, in shops, cinemas, leisure facilities, etc.

- Parents have to cope with a variety of life situations balanced against their child's demand for sweets, chocolate and biscuits, testing a parent's patience and ability to withstand these requests.

- Parents' lack of knowledge of the sugar content in the foods their child eats, along with any long-term danger to health as a result.

Matt says, 'Our six-year-old son was always a nightmare on shopping trips or on days out because his focus was on sweets or a sugary drink or ice cream. It got to the stage where we would take it in turns to stay at home with him while the other one did the shopping and we stopped going out on family trips to avoid the drama. He would scream in the supermarket aisles, lay on the floor and refuse to move, grab sweets off the shelves and put them in the trolley or eat them there and then – all while people around us looked on thinking we were bad parents. My wife then decided to look into why he might be behaving that way and she found from her research that it was down to sugar in the diet and changes in blood glucose. Our son was having too much sugar from fizzy drinks and biscuits, more or less on demand. We made very gradual changes to wean him off the bad stuff, replacing these foods with healthier alternatives. We no longer buy sugary drinks, snacks, children's yoghurts, etc. Eight months on, I'm happy to say that our son is now a well-behaved child and we can take him anywhere without the tantrums.'

In order to help parents reduce their child's sugar intake, the Government could take further action in the following ways:

- Introduce a ban on confectionery and fizzy drinks vending machines in schools.

- Increase availability and access to more free weight management courses with subsidies at swimming pools and sports facilities for young people.

- Tax all high-sugar foods and subsidise healthy foods for children.

- Impose laws regarding a reduction in the amount of sugar, salt and fat that manufacturers add to food.

- Enable parents to choose healthier options for their children's meals with clearer food labelling.

- Introduce media health education messages about obesity in childhood and the development of associated health problems.

- Local councils reduce the number of fast-food restaurants near schools and encourage local restaurants and cafés to offer healthier food choices.

Some of the above are already taking shape and it is hoped that many, if not all of these measures will be adopted in the near future.

Why manufacturers add sugar to foods

We are eating more and more foods containing sugar. Millions of pounds are spent on advertising these foods every year to compel us to buy them. Manufacturers add inexpensive and versatile sugars to recipes in numerous ways to bulk them up, add flavour, colour or to increase shelf-life. Children in the UK are exposed to a high volume of marketing and advertising in various ways including TV advertising, radio, cinema, press and billboards, social media and online advertising, as well as via food and drinks manufacturers' sponsorship of TV programmes, public events and amenities. Research has shown that all types of marketing and publicity consistently influence food preference, choice and purchasing in children and adults.

According to Public Health England, food price promotions are more widespread in the UK than in any other country in Europe.

Foods on promotion account for around 40 per cent of all spending on food and drinks consumed at home, with products containing a high amount of sugar being promoted more than other foods. These supermarket price promotions increase the amount of food and drink people buy by around one-fifth and these are purchases people often do not intend to make without in-store promotions. Impulse buys also increase the amount of higher-sugar foods and drinks purchased by 6 per cent overall, influencing purchasing by all socio-economic and demographic groups.

FACT: _____

A crackdown on junk-food advertisements would help to tackle the current childhood obesity epidemic.

A person's sugar intake is dependent on several things:

- Influencers from marketing and advertising campaigns and product promotions encouraging us to purchase and consume the product.

- Availability of the food or drink for purchase, for example supermarkets and other food retail outlets, cafés and restaurants as well as food and drink available in the workplace and school canteens.

- Knowledge, training and education to enable healthy food choices concerning the risks associated with consuming too much sugar.

As I've mentioned previously, Public Health England advises certain restrictions on sugar consumption for children, although no amount of sugar is 'safe' to eat. It is important to keep sugar intake as low as possible. PHE recommendations for children's sugar consumption are as follows:

Age	Maximum sugar intake	Equivalent sugar cubes	Equivalent teaspoons
4–6 years	No more than 19g per day	5 cubes	4–5 teaspoons
7–10 years	No more than 24g per day	6 cubes	5–6 teaspoons
11 years plus	No more than 30g per day	7 cubes	6–7 teaspoons

The UK is a world leader in diet and health for areas such as lowering salt consumption, action in schools to improve the nutrition of food provided, and imposing strict criteria on TV advertising to children. Action to reduce sugar consumption is the next key concern. It is likely that added sugars will be highlighted separately on food labels in the near future.

In September 2019, Public Health England announced that manufacturers' efforts to reduce the amount of added sugar in foods by 5 per cent still had a long way to go. Between 2015 and 2018, the average sugar content of shop-bought food fell by only 2.9 per cent, while the amount of sugar we consume had increased despite the sugar tax on soft drinks, although these products now contain 29 per cent less sugar. Manufacturers have stated that a 5 per cent reduction in added sugar is too ambitious.

Where does sugar come from?

The vast majority of the sugar we consume comes from sugar cane or beet. Sugar beet and sugar cane have equal sweetness as both contain 99.9 per cent pure sucrose. Cane sugar has been cultivated for 2,500 years, originating in China and India and spreading west until, by the sixteenth century, it had reached the Caribbean. Raw sugar was then shipped to Europe to be refined. Originally, cane sugar referred to the juice squeezed from sugar cane although the majority of sugar today is refined white sugar.

Processing sugar cane involves boiling it several times to

produce both cane sugar and raw molasses (syrup). After it is processed again, the remaining molasses contain very little sugar and what is left at this final stage is used for cattle food or to make yeast. Each stage of boiling causes the raw sugar to change colour: pale brown sugar is called demerara; darker brown sugar from the second boiling is called light muscovado; after the third boiling the sugar is darkest and is known as dark muscovado. The final stage is for the sugar to be refined into white sugar by washing it.

FACT: _____

'Plantation white' sugar is formed when sugar cane juice is chemically treated.

Sugar beet is a white root related to beetroot and chard; the production process is less involved than with sugar cane as the molasses from sugar beet are unpalatable, while the juice is processed in the same way as cane sugar. Fifty per cent of sugar produced in the UK comes from sugar cane and 50 per cent from sugar beet. Sugar manufacture has risen steadily over the years so that we now produce in excess of 100,000 tons per annum and, over the past century, there has been a twenty-five-fold rise in world sugar production.

Types of sugar

White sugar (refined cane or beet sugar):
granulated; caster; cubed; preserving

Raw sugar (unrefined cane sugar):
golden granulated raw cane; Demerara raw cane;
Dark muscovado raw cane

Brown sugar (refined white cane/beet sugar plus molasses):
light soft brown; dark soft brown

TIP: _____

If you feel you cannot give up all sugar in tea, coffee and home baking, using high-quality dark muscovado sugar with a high molasses content is a good compromise. Dark muscovado sugar, with a greater amount of molasses, has some nutritional content.

_____

Raw cane sugar is a mixture of sugar cane and white cane sugar, so it cannot be defined as pure and natural; equally, refined white sugar becomes impure because it has been processed and is not in its original state. Much of the brown sugar we buy is coloured with molasses or caramel. Brown sugar that has been coloured in this way is similar to white sugar and has no nutritional value because the quantity of added molasses is small.

The amount of sugar in our food

Sugar is an indispensable substance to manufacturers because it has so many properties besides adding immediate sweetness to food and drink. Sugar is also used as a flavour enhancer in savoury foods like sauces, soups, vegetables, coffee and some processed meats. It interacts with certain flavours to make them more intense. Used as a preservative, sugar prevents decay and mould forming in foods such as jam and marmalade, as well as helping them set by enabling the action of pectin. It provides texture in sweet foods and can be used to decorate cakes or caramelise savoury foods like bread crust or onions. Sugar absorbs water, which is good for food preservation and provides bulk to foods like yoghurts, extending shelf-life. Sugar makes soft drinks taste full-bodied over their diet, low-sugar counterparts. Sugar feeds yeast in the fermentation process during wine production. Because sugar has so many uses in the manufacturing of food we are consuming more and more of it. This increases the degree by which sugar can cause varying effects on the body. While manufacturers justify the use of sugar in foods for the above reasons, the reality is that significant amounts of sugar are being added to almost all processed foods.

FACT: _____

Current estimates of UK sugar intake from the National Diet and Nutrition Survey programme show that school-aged children and teenagers are eating three times more sugar every day than is recommended; adults are consuming around twice the maximum recommended level of sugar per day.

The brain uses more energy than any other organ in the human body and glucose is its primary source of fuel, although eating more sugar to be turned into glucose doesn't result in better brain function. Every time blood glucose is elevated above normal limits it is harmful to the brain, resulting in slowed mental function and lapses in memory and attention. Food manufacturers have realised that children like sweet things and that they are more likely to eat something if it tastes sweet. Manufacturers also know that sugar is an addictive substance. Children should eat the same foods that adults eat, not breakfast cereals specifically aimed at children's love of sugary food.

A recent study looked at fizzy drink consumption in six schools in the UK and 644 schoolchildren aged between seven and eleven over one school year.[5] Half the children had been told they could improve their health by avoiding fizzy drinks while the other half were only told that having a healthy lifestyle involves regular exercise and eating less fat. At the end of the school year the percentage of overweight children had increased by 7.5 per cent for the children that had been told to exercise and reduce the amount of fat in their diet. The children who had reduced their daily intake of fizzy drinks by half a glass – 125ml – had reduced their weight by an average 7.7 per cent by comparison, showing that the health education received about sugar consumption had a positive effect.

Fourteen-year-old twins Joanne and Leanne say, 'We had a lesson on healthy eating at school and it really helped us realise about unhealthy choices. We used to buy a can of fizzy drink on the way to school and again on the way home. The lesson explained the calories in sugary drinks and that over a year, that was the same as having 78,000 extra calories with no nutrition, leading to weight gain. We've now swapped to sugar-free drinks and they really do taste better, plus being healthier.'

A second study in the journal of Public Health Nutrition[6] examining the amount of salt and sugar added to children's breakfast cereals showed that while the level of salt had decreased from 1992 to 2015 in the UK, levels of sugar have remained consistently high. A suggested portion size of 30g of sweet cereal contains, on average, one-third of the recommended daily amount of sugar for a four- to six-year-old in the UK – 19g. Have a look for the different sugars in the foods you have in your own kitchen and get children to join in. Here's a list of sugars that manufacturers add to the food we eat:

agave syrup	fruit juice	microcrystalline
barley malt	concentrate	cellulose
beet sugar	galactose	molasses
brown rice sugar	glucose	polydextrose
brown sugar	granulated sugar	powdered sugar
cane juice	high-fructose corn	raisin juice
confectioner's	syrup	(fructose)
sugar	honey	raisin syrup
corn sweetener	invert sugar	raw sugar
corn syrup	lactose	sorbitol
date sugar	maltodextrin	Sucanat
dextrin	malted barley	sucrose
dextrose	maltitol	sugar cane
fructooliosacharides	maltose	turbinado sugar
fructose	mannitol	white sugar
	maple sugar	xylitol

You may have been persuaded by manufacturers that some of these sugars are healthier because they are natural and derived from honey or fruit. Always remember that sugar is sugar and as such, it will increase blood glucose levels when it is broken down in the digestive system. If more than one of the above sugars is listed on an ingredients label then that food is very high in added sugar.

TIP:

Always read food labels before you buy to assess the amount of sugar and glucose added to what you eat and what you give your family at mealtimes. Avoid foods with more than one type of added sugar.

Baby formula is made from dried cow's milk with the addition of increased sweetness from honey or fruit sources rather than the less-sweet lactose, the natural sugar found in milk. It is easy to see that with manufacturers of baby milk adding sugars in this way, babies are introduced to sweeter foods very early on in their lives and this desire for sweet, comforting food and drink stays with them. As children grow they are given cereals and fruit with added sugar, such as canned fruit in syrup rather than fresh fruit, and later biscuits, chocolate and sweets. A child is not born wanting sugar; it is offered to them and they develop a taste for it, which becomes a craving.

FACT:

When manufacturers produce foods that are labelled 'low fat', the sugar content is increased to enhance the flavour lost from reducing the amount of fat. Remember: low fat equals higher sugar.

Sugar is added to the foods we buy from restaurants and manufacturers to make them taste nice. Even savoury foods such as sauces, soups, baked beans, pickle, pickled onions, ketchup, vegetables, tinned meat, peanut butter, tomato juice, snacks and convenience foods have sugar added to them in the production process. Certain foods and drinks are marketed as energy-boosting. This is not the case, as all food provides the body with energy. Energy cannot be instantly increased by eating sugar: dietary sugar is converted into glucose and stored for use by the muscles when it's needed. The exception is in the case of low blood glucose levels in children and adults with diabetes and people who experience low blood glucose when they haven't eaten for several hours. Sugar is then absorbed by the stomach lining to raise blood glucose levels back to normal quickly. For people without diabetes who need an energy boost, eat a banana rather than having a glucose or high-sugar drink or eating confectionery, cakes and biscuits. Despite what the food industry tells us – that sugar is vital because it provides us with instant energy – sugar is not necessary in the diet.

FACT:

Foods and drinks with a high sugar content are marketed as boosting energy quickly because they have no other value. It is worth remembering that eating sugar or glucose causes insulin to be released to reduce blood glucose levels again, possibly to a lower level than before consuming the food or drink.

Sugar is praised for being pure. In the sense that it is produced in such a way that what is left at the end of the process is chemically pure, this is true. However, in terms of consuming something that is pure, meaning risk-free or beneficial to the body, this is not the case. When sugary foods and drinks become too large a part of a normal diet, this leads to poor nutrition. It is possible to consume 500 calories or more a day just by adding sugar to tea or coffee and breakfast cereal: a heaped teaspoon of sugar is 30 calories. If this figure is added to the calories and sugar content in things like ice cream, biscuits and chocolate, this total from 'empty calories' provides little nutritional value. Because these foods taste good, they are more likely to be consumed.

KEY MESSAGES IN THIS CHAPTER

- The UK Government introduced the Soft Drinks Industry Levy (SDIL) in April 2018 as part of its childhood obesity strategy. This tax puts a charge of 24p on drinks containing 8g of sugar per 100ml and 18p a litre on those with 5–8g of sugar per 100ml.

- Public Health England suggest that adults and children over the age of eleven should have no more than 30g of sugar per day and that sugar should make up no more than 5 per cent of daily calories.

- Evidence shows that slowly changing the amount of sugar, salt and fat in foods, or reducing product size, is a successful way to make products healthier.

- There has been an average 11 per cent reduction in sugar and 6 per cent average calories per portion for retailers' own-label brands and manufacturers' private-label products.

- Be aware of what you're eating. Always check the list of ingredients on foods before you buy, even if you don't think they appear sweet. The ingredients are listed by weight, so those at the beginning are present in the greatest amounts – words like 'glucose' or 'syrup' indicate high-sugar foods.

- Using high-quality dark muscovado sugar with a high molasses content is preferable when you're reducing the family's sugar intake as it has some nutritional content.

- Children and teenagers are eating three times more sugar every day than is recommended; adults are consuming around twice the maximum recommended level of sugar per day.

Sugar and Health Issues

We know that eating too much sugar is bad for us because it can have a negative effect on the body. Sugary drinks, confectionery, sweet baked goods and sweetened dairy products remain the chief source of added sugars in the diet of adults and children, providing little or no nutritional value. To make things worse, these added sugars can be difficult to find on food labels as they are often listed under different names, like maltodextrin or fruit juice concentrate. All of these added sugars can affect the health of you and your family in a number of different ways that will be explained in more detail in this chapter.

How dietary sugars are processed by the body

A high-sugar diet affects every bodily system because blood glucose reaches every part of the body. When food is eaten it is processed by the digestive system. Nutrients and toxins are extracted during this process to pass directly into the blood where they are chemically transformed and filtered. Useful substances are stored or used in the body while unnecessary substances are detoxified. This process is ongoing and when harmful substances are metabolised in the body, the liver is the primary organ to be affected.

When a person's diet is high in sugar, the liver becomes enlarged, partly because fat cells increase in number and in size. Sugar consumption causes fibrous scar tissue to form in the liver, something that is normally seen in people who have chronic alcoholism and associated cirrhosis of the liver. The scar tissue is made of collagen, which is the protein that is present in the walls of the body cells, forming the major part of connective tissue, tendons and ligaments. Sugar is known to increase the amount of collagen formed by the body – something that is observed in people with diabetes. In turn, this can cause joints to become stiff and ligaments and tendons to shorten.

FACT: _____

A high-sugar diet can lead to an increase in the size of the kidneys and the adrenal glands that sit on top of them. A high-sugar diet has been shown to increase the production of adrenal hormone by up to 400 per cent.

Eating too many free sugars – sugars added to food and drinks in the home or by manufacturers, plus sugars that are naturally present in food – increases the total calories consumed as part of the diet, leading to weight gain for adults and children. Being overweight increases the risk of developing heart disease, Type 2 diabetes, stroke and certain types of cancer. Obesity is a major health issue: in 2012, 25 per cent of adults were classed as obese, while almost 40 per cent were overweight.[1] Weight gain in children is a particular concern. In 2012, 10 per cent of four- to five-year-olds and almost 20 per cent of children aged ten to eleven years were classed as obese.[2] By 2017, 30 per cent of children aged two to fifteen in England were overweight or obese, including 17 per cent who were obese.[3] Studies have also shown that excessive sugar intake leads to tooth decay, especially in children. In 2013, 33 per cent of children aged five years and almost 50 per cent of eight-year-olds had decay in their milk teeth, with 34 per cent of children aged twelve and almost half of fifteen-year-olds having tooth decay. In 2014, a survey of three-year-olds found that 12 per cent had visible tooth decay, with on average three affected teeth.[4]

High blood glucose levels

Glucose enters the bloodstream, travelling to the muscles and powering bodily functions. This situation is fine if any excess glucose is used by the body during exercise, but the natural response to a high glucose level in a child or adult without Type 1 diabetes is for insulin to be released by the pancreas. Insulin then does its job of reducing blood glucose levels to make them normal again.

When starches are consumed – wholegrain bread, wholewheat pasta or potatoes – blood glucose levels are steadily maintained because these foods do not cause sudden spikes in the amount of glucose available. This is not the case if foods containing a high amount of glucose or free sugar are eaten because a large amount of insulin is produced to deal with the sudden rush of glucose, and this can reduce blood glucose levels to the opposite extreme. The 'sugar rush' can cause mood swings, headaches and tiredness because blood glucose levels become too low. The body reacts by making us feel hungry again – craving sweet foods – in order to boost flagging blood glucose levels, so more food is eaten, leading to weight gain.

After eating a high-sugar diet for just two weeks, the fasting blood glucose level – the level measured when no food and just water has been taken for eight hours – contains 40 per cent more glucose when compared with someone who eats a low-sugar diet. By eating a healthy, low-sugar diet you can avoid this blood glucose yo-yo effect, reducing the likelihood of weight gain, mood swings and tiredness. A key issue here for adults and children is the future development of Type 2 diabetes, which is now being diagnosed in children as young as three years of age, because more insulin has to be produced when the body struggles to maintain normal blood glucose levels.

Experiments have shown that research subjects fed a high-sugar diet for a couple of weeks became intolerant to sugar and required more insulin to reduce blood glucose levels.[5] Their body tissues had adapted to high sugar consumption and eventually became unable to cope with the increased blood glucose levels it caused, while a low-sugar diet for a couple of weeks reversed this situation.

FACT: _____

Compared to an adult, a child is far more sensitive to a sharp rise or fall in blood glucose.

Low blood glucose levels

Low blood glucose levels make both children and adults feel hungry and weak. A person with low blood glucose levels may experience sweating and shaking, with dizziness and a bad headache. If blood glucose levels are not raised quickly, mental confusion occurs with slurred speech. This can happen when a carbohydrate-rich meal or snack is eaten, causing a large amount of insulin to be released by the pancreas to deal with the associated rise in blood glucose. Fat and protein will also be converted into glucose at this time – for example, after eating a fast-food meal with a high starch and sugar content – but glucose from protein and fat metabolism is produced at a slower pace.

Excess blood glucose is converted into glycogen and stored in the liver and muscles. If a great deal of glucose is stored in this way – after eating sugary snacks between meals, for example – then absorption is slow and the blood glucose level remains high. It is easy to see how erratic blood glucose levels can occur in this way when eating high-sugar foods.

To prevent such dramatic fluctuations in blood glucose levels it is important for children and adults to eat foods that raise blood glucose levels slowly and evenly, such as porridge oats or wholegrain bread. Babies can be especially prone to developing low blood glucose levels because they are unable to maintain a normal blood glucose-insulin balance. In extreme cases, this can cause unconsciousness when the blood glucose level falls very low (hypoglycaemia); in such emergency situations, medical professionals will treat hypoglycaemia using intravenous glucose.

Behavioural and emotional issues

As we have already seen, carbohydrates are broken down into sugars by the body and used for energy. When we eat carbohydrates such as wholewheat pasta, potatoes or brown rice, these foods provide a steady source of energy. When we eat something like a doughnut or pancakes with syrup, the energy release is very rapid because these foods contain a high level of sugar. The body reacts to an energy hit by producing insulin to reduce blood glucose levels back down to normal. This reduction may be sudden, causing a feeling of tiredness, weakness and headache.

To put the effects of erratic blood glucose levels for a non-diabetic child into a real-life situation, imagine this scenario: a child has crisps and Coke on the way to school with friends, causing a sugar rush when reaching school for 09:00. The insulin response to the sugar in the Coke means that by 10:30 in the morning, the child's blood glucose will have dropped down again, possibly on the lower side of normal with associated mood swings, tiredness and an inability to concentrate in class. If the child then eats a lunch causing a rapid increase in blood glucose again – which they will crave because blood glucose levels are low, there will be a rapid increase in blood glucose followed by another low, making the child feel sluggish and tired during afternoon lessons.

The sudden fall in blood glucose in response to eating something very sweet is not the same as low blood glucose in people with diabetes, where glucose levels may fall below normal limits where the brain can't function normally. It's not only an unstable blood glucose level that the body has to deal with when there is a peak and then rapid drop in blood glucose. The body also releases adrenaline when blood glucose drops quickly to protect the brain from becoming starved of glucose for fuel. If this is the situation long-term, the body rebels, becoming easily fatigued. Adults and children who eat a lot of sugar tend to be fixated on getting more sugar because it makes them feel better, allowing them to focus in the short term on the task at hand. Research has shown that a dependency on any substance adversely affects the way we have relationships with others.

Paula, a children's nurse, says, 'My son Ben is ten and we experienced years of behaviour issues before we cut sugar from the family diet. To assess if your child's behaviour is related to sugar, ask a few simple questions about sugar habits like, does your child frequently crave sweet foods? Are there monumental tantrums if they don't get what they want? Does your child have regular episodes of hyperactivity with trouble sleeping? Have you seen your child suddenly change temperament – a joy to be with one minute and stroppy the next? If the answer to any of these questions is 'yes', your child has erratic blood glucose swings because of sugar in their diet. You may have already realised that some behaviours get worse after your child drinks a Coke or eats sugary cereal for breakfast but you know they enjoy it and you can't see how to stop your child having these foods.'

As a parent, it is important to know that behaviour related to high or low blood glucose levels is not the fault of you or your child.

Attention Deficit Hyperactivity Disorder (ADHD)

Children diagnosed with Attention Deficit Hyperactivity Disorder may have difficulty processing information and they may also be prescribed medication to help decrease ADHD symptoms. A high-sugar diet will make this condition worse because sugar calms the brain, allowing the child to concentrate and be relaxed for a short period. This causes them to rely on sugar, meaning that when they need a sugar hit they can become argumentative and irritable until their craving is satisfied. A child's activity level and their sugar intake has been described as 'reverse causality' – where very active children need more energy derived from starches and sugars to fuel that activity, so they seek out sugary foods to provide a 'fast hit' of sugar as a result.

FACT: _____

Research has suggested that hyperactivity in children is due to an excess of dietary sugar and that the condition can be reversed or vastly improved with a low-sugar diet if sugar cannot be removed from the diet completely.[6]

High-sugar snacks can cause your child to become hyperactive because digesting them requires the pancreas to secrete a large amount of insulin, which ultimately lowers their blood glucose levels. This stimulates an increase in the hormone epinephrine, triggering nervous reactions and hyperactivity disorder behaviours. Studies have shown that a diet high in sugary snacks increases the likelihood of nutritional imbalance, lower emotional intelligence and ADHD.[7] Recent research on dietary sugar has suggested that higher consumption of sugar is positively linked with an increased level of hyperactivity and attention deficiency similar to ADHD.[8] While some specialists believe a high-sugar diet is a causal factor of ADHD in association with a lack of proper nutrition, others do not.

FACT: _____

Children who consume 600–700 calories per day from sugary snacks are at greater risk of developing or worsening ADHD behaviours.

If your child often has temper tantrums that are calmed by eating something sweet, they may be diagnosed with hyperactivity or Attention Deficit Disorder (ADD) because the child is addicted to sugar. The gradual introduction of a low-sugar diet over several months or even longer should result in improvements. You know your child best, which will allow you to judge whether they still have behavioural problems after reducing their sugar intake over the long term. I'm not suggesting that everything can be cured with a low-sugar diet, but many parents have reported that their child no longer has trouble paying attention after making this lifestyle change.

Danielle says, 'When my daughter was diagnosed with ADHD her consultant was adamant that diet played no part in her behaviour. She was prescribed Ritalin and took it for ten months. I then looked on the Internet and found that some studies agreed with the consultant while others suggested that dietary sugar could play a part in behaviour. I took the matter into my own hands and began cutting sugar from my daughter's diet. Although she was still taking the prescribed medication, once I removed as much sugar as possible from her diet her behaviour was like flicking a switch: there were fewer and fewer hyperactive episodes over the weeks and now, after six months of low sugar, none. I'm going to report this massive improvement to the consultant at our next appointment and ask him if my daughter can come off the Ritalin.'

Altered hormone levels

Hormones are chemical messengers in the body that help to control nearly every physiological process such as metabolism, the proper functioning of your immune system and your reproductive system. Imbalances in hormone levels can lead to health conditions.

Hormonal balance is crucial to health because if one hormone level is altered, this adversely affects the function of other hormones and when this happens the body compensates by enhancing or restricting production to correct the imbalance. This happens naturally during puberty, pregnancy and the menopause. Throughout the various stages of life, hormones are naturally in flux. However, hormone levels may be adversely affected due to lifestyle factors such as increased stress, not getting enough sleep or exercise, and high levels of fat and sugar in the diet. While it may not be easy to reduce the level of stress in your life or increase the amount of sleep you get, reducing the amount of dietary sugar is something we can all do to have a significant effect on improving the levels and function of several hormones.

It is important to reduce dietary sugar intake for many

beneficial reasons, not just for the effect sugar has on body weight. For females especially, a diet high in added sugars from refined carbohydrates can cause significant hormonal imbalance leading, for example, to insulin resistance, a precursor to Type 2 diabetes. Insulin, the hormone that stops blood glucose levels from rising too high, is constantly fluctuating due to dietary glucose and other factors, sending many different signals throughout the body to process and use the energy we get from carbohydrate. Once insulin resistance develops due to a high-sugar diet, the muscles, fat and liver cells change the way they respond to insulin. Insulin resistance is a complex metabolic issue which can eventually lead to serious conditions like Type 2 diabetes, obesity, high levels of cholesterol (blood fats), heart disease and even stroke.

A high-sugar diet can have significant effects on the reproductive hormones. When more and more insulin is being produced to reduce blood glucose levels after eating something sweet (insulin resistance), the symptoms of polycystic ovary syndrome (PCOS) can change and worsen over time. PCOS symptoms may include acne, weight gain or difficulty losing weight, excess hair on the face and body, irregular periods, fertility problems and depression. Most women with PCOS will experience insulin resistance as it is the most common physiological imbalance associated with the condition.

Although it is often claimed that children now reach puberty earlier than they did a century ago due to a more nutritious diet, research has shown that it is the amount of sugar in the modern diet that causes children to reach sexual maturity at an earlier age due to the effect sugar has on hormonal levels.[9]

Eating too much fructose and glucose can turn off the gene that regulates the body's levels of active testosterone and oestrogen, oestrogen being responsible for a number of processes in the body, such as regulating the reproductive system as well as helping boost the action of insulin. When reducing sugar in the diet of younger female children, PCOS is obviously not an issue. However, signs of hormonal imbalance and physical and emotional symptoms will present in other ways, such as sleep disorders, fatigue, mood changes, difficulty concentrating, feeling irritable and low mood.

TIP:

Plant foods such as soy that contain phytoestrogens – groups of chemicals that act in a similar way to oestrogen in the body – may help address many health conditions. Flaxseed is another significant source of phytoestrogens, which can help promote hormone balance if taken regularly.

Serotonin is another hormone affected by blood glucose levels. Children who have unstable blood glucose levels that drop regularly also have low serotonin levels – the hormone that calms the brain – making the child feel edgy and less able to deal with stress.[10]

When we consider that dietary carbohydrate (starch) is broken down into sugar by the body and the effects sugar has on hormone levels, it is unsurprising that children today are not only growing taller, they are developing weight problems and health conditions previously only seen in adults such as sleep apnoea and Type 2 diabetes. A diet that is made up of lots of refined carbohydrates and processed foods is the most common contributor to insulin resistance and hormonal imbalance. Make changes by avoiding these foods wherever possible and try to include a variety of organic vegetables and fruits, whole grains, low-fat dairy products and lean sources of protein, such as fish, in your family's diet. Caffeine consumption from coffee and cola drinks should also be avoided or significantly reduced, as these can disrupt cortisol hormones. Cortisol helps control blood glucose levels, regulates metabolism, helps reduce inflammation and assists with memory formulation. Cortisol also has a controlling effect on salt and water balance in the body and helps control blood pressure.

TIP: _____

Reducing sugar in the diet will go a long way towards improving hormone imbalance. As it has taken many years to develop and adapt the diet you now eat with many changes along the way, reducing foods containing sugar and swapping high-sugar foods for healthier options will take time too.

Hereditary Fructose Disorder in babies

Fructose is fruit sugar, twice as sweet as sucrose or glucose and naturally found in honey, maple syrup and agave syrup from the agave plant. Fructose is often used to sweeten diabetic foods as it does not raise blood glucose levels in the same way that glucose does, although fructose can be indigestible, causing hereditary fructose intolerance in babies. This is a rare genetic condition that is caused by a deficiency of the enzyme aldolase B, which metabolises fructose. This disorder can be particularly concerning in babies as it causes blood glucose levels to plummet and dangerous substances to build up in the liver.

Individuals affected with hereditary fructose intolerance will show no symptoms until they eat a food containing fructose, sucrose or sorbitol. If fructose is ingested, the enzyme error causes an accumulation of fructose-1-phosphate which, over time, results in the death of liver cells. After eating fructose, individuals with hereditary fructose intolerance may experience nausea, bloating, abdominal pain, diarrhoea, vomiting and low blood glucose levels – hypoglycaemia. Treatment of the condition involves eliminating fructose and sucrose from the diet. When hereditary fructose intolerance is severe, removing these sugars from the diet may not be enough to prevent progressive liver disease.

Type 1 diabetes

Type 1 diabetes develops most often in children and young adults, although people in their twenties, thirties and older can also be diagnosed with this condition. Type 1 diabetes is a form of diabetes in which the insulin-producing cells of the pancreas stop working because they are destroyed by the body's immune system. Insulin, which controls blood glucose levels in the body, has to be replaced by injection instead. This type of diabetes is not caused by obesity or lifestyle factors and it cannot be reversed. Eating a low-sugar diet, however, makes Type 1 diabetes very much easier to manage, as it helps keep blood glucose levels stable. I can testify to this fact as I've had Type 1 diabetes since childhood. It is important for people with Type 1 diabetes to manage blood glucose levels well at all times so they don't become too high or fall too low. If low blood glucose (hypoglycaemia) occurs, glucose is necessary.

Obesity in children and adults

Children require a certain number of calories per day for building new cells so they can grow and function. Toddlers use half of their daily calorie intake for brain function alone, with the remainder used for growth; requirements for brain function increase to 65 per cent of daily calories for a two-year-old. By age ten, children require 2,000 calories a day, the same amount as an adult female. Hormones are released to tell us when we need to eat food and again to tell us when we are full and should stop eating. However, if the blood contains a raised level of cholesterol and triglycerides (fats) the hormones that signal when we are full work less effectively, so we tend to eat more. By eating a diet high in sugary snacks and drinks, children and adults can become overweight.

The effects of a modern diet and busy lifestyle are present in young children who develop high blood fat and glucose levels and the health problems that go with it. In South America in 2017, a baby boy was found to be so overweight he had already developed Type 2 diabetes, high blood pressure and fatty liver disease: his mother fed him on demand and he was always hungry.[11]

FACT: _____

One in four children leaving school is considered obese. There are currently 1.2 million obese children in the UK and a hundred children every year are diagnosed with Type 2 diabetes.

Weight gain occurs because calories are consumed above the amount needed to fuel the body. It is unlikely that a child or adult would gain weight because they are eating too much meat, fish or fresh fruit; the parts of the diet that increase body weight are those with the most calories eaten most often, such as crisps, non-diet fizzy drinks, cakes and biscuits. Sugar that is added to baby formula and cereal given to infants leads to excessive weight gain; the childhood obesity epidemic in the UK is testament to this problem. Just like adults, babies and children gain weight if they consume more calories than they need.

Individuals who add 500 daily calories or more of sugar to foods and drinks such as tea, coffee and breakfast cereals may reduce their consumption of nutritious food during the day to compensate for this. However, this is not usually the case – instead the foods and drinks containing added sugar are consumed on top of the rest of their diet and this becomes the norm. If one's diet contains 2,500 calories a day, of which 500 calories come from sugar, then one-fifth of the daily calorie intake provides no nutritional value at all. When sugar is consumed, the body will either use it for energy or it will store the sugar as fat for later use. If you've ever thought you had gained weight from eating too many high-fat foods over the holidays, the reality is that this excess weight was down to sugar storage.

Jill says, 'I've always struggled with my weight and so have my children. I have a nine-year-old and an eleven-year-old and they were hooked on biscuits, cakes, sweets, etc., and if I'm honest, so was I. I was setting an example to them by buying those things from the supermarket because I wanted to show love, only instead I was setting them up for a lifetime of being overweight with potential health problems. Luckily, a friend who is a nutritionist told me to cut the sugar from our diets, making wanting to improve my children's health my main motivation. It worked and I can truly say that by reading labels carefully and cutting out processed, sugary foods, we've all lost weight without consciously dieting. We all eat a healthy, balanced diet now and we've each lost several kilos. It's like a no-brainer but I never made the connection between eating sweet foods and not being able to lose weight because many famous diets say you can eat the foods you love – like chocolate and desserts – and still lose weight if you count calories or points. That way, you never get over craving sugar and you are not having a healthy diet.'

If you have an overweight child or you've struggled all your life to keep your weight under control, cutting sugar as part of a lifestyle change can be the answer. I can personally attest to this, losing 7.5kg by eating a healthy diet and swapping to reduced sugar options of sauces and soups and this weight has stayed off with the continuation of a low-sugar diet, requiring me to take less insulin. Don't forget, insulin enables fat to be stored in the body and excess sugar is stored as fat too. The approach many people with Type 1 diabetes have taken has been that you can eat freely as long as you give yourself the correct amount of insulin to cover the blood glucose increase for that food. However, a low-sugar diet means that less insulin is needed and you can maintain a steady blood glucose level and weight, all of which are hugely important for better health.

A low-sugar lifestyle is not about adopting a calorie-controlled, restrictive diet; it's about healthy, sensible eating – making good food choices rather than sugary ones. High-sugar foods and drinks tend to be high in calories so cut these out and replace them with better alternatives. By also incorporating some exercise into your family routine you will spend time together walking or cycling, helping you lose weight and feel fitter because you have made a positive lifestyle change. This is not about denial and dieting; it's about finding healthier alternatives.

If your child is trying to lose weight and you've begun the gradual removal of sugars from the family diet, it's also advisable to cut back on excess calories from fried foods and high-fat savoury snacks too. While a lifestyle change isn't a diet, weight loss will only be achieved and sustained if other changes are made that help the process – like replacing fried food with grilled food. However, it's important that growing children have good fats in their diet from sources such as tuna, mackerel and salmon. Consider swapping higher-fat proteins in your child's diet such as peanut butter or cheese for ones like lean ham, eggs or skinless chicken as most of the fat is found under the skin.

TIP: _____

If you can't stretch your budget to tuna, mackerel or salmon, give your child a cod-liver oil capsule to take with their breakfast to provide essential omega-3 fatty acids for brain development.

_____

Obesity is not always due to eating too much of the wrong types of food; it may be due to insulin resistance which, as I mentioned earlier, is another name for pre-diabetes. If blood glucose is continually elevated and this glucose cannot be used for fuel because insulin can't work properly, the excess glucose gets converted into stored fat. This means that two different children might eat the same foods but because one has insulin resistance, they will gain more weight than the other child. The more fat that is stored in the body cells, the harder it is for insulin to work properly to bring down blood glucose levels, which results in that glucose being stored as more fat. If your family adopts a low-sugar lifestyle, this circle is broken and once weight starts to be lost, insulin has a better opportunity to work. This is the basis of reversing Type 2 diabetes by reducing body weight, allowing insulin to do its job properly.

FACT: _____

Obesity is not caused by a lack of willpower and it is not a choice. Making children and adults feel ashamed if they have a weight problem – known as fat shaming – will make them feel worse. Support is necessary to enable lifestyle change.

Moving around uses up more calories than sitting still. Certain popular activities involve sitting for long periods of time without moving much, computer gaming and watching hours of TV being prime examples. Make it a game with your children to add up the amount of time spent doing these activities every day and every week. If the answer shocks you, suggest a gradual change to more physical exercise – going to play outside on their bikes, for example. If you have the time, you could join in. Don't cut TV and computer games completely; introduce a more sensible limit so they don't miss their favourite TV shows, but they're not staring at the screen for hours.

Type 2 diabetes in children and adults

Type 2 is the most common form of diabetes, affecting around 90 per cent of people with diabetes around the world. It is usually caused by lifestyle factors, although it can also occur in older people when insulin works less efficiently. This condition is most often associated with obesity, especially around the waistline and abdomen, and a lack of regular exercise. A high intake of dietary sugars has not been shown to cause Type 2 diabetes directly, but this can lead to obesity which is a major risk factor for the development of the condition. Recommendations for people with Type 2 diabetes include weight loss and altering one's lifestyle to eat a healthy diet. These recommendations are the same for the rest of the population: we should all eat a healthy diet and take regular exercise.

Type 2 diabetes in adults and children is a complex condition that begins when the body stops responding to insulin because it's unable to work well in the presence of excess fat cells. With Type 2 diabetes, more and more insulin is needed to bring blood glucose levels under control and this creates a condition known as insulin resistance. The insulin that is made by the body is unable to enter the cells to allow glucose to be burned as fuel for energy. When an adult or child eats a high-sugar diet including lots of refined carbohydrates that don't take much breaking down to extract their energy, blood glucose levels rise rapidly and stay high as more sugary foods keep the blood glucose level abnormally raised. This means that there is a toxic level of glucose in the blood and other hormones then struggle to work properly when there is this imbalance of insulin. Eating a low-sugar diet and taking regular exercise are major steps to avoiding obesity and the development of Type 2 diabetes.

Eyesight

Eye specialists have long reported the association between high blood glucose levels and damage to the retina at the back of the eyes in people with diabetes. Eye disease due to higher than normal blood glucose levels is less common in children before their teenage years. However, eating a high-sugar diet that frequently causes spikes in blood glucose levels damages the tiny blood vessels at the back of the eyes in both diabetic and non-diabetic children and adults, with the potential to cause sight problems.

As we have already seen, a high-sugar diet causes metabolic dysfunction leading to weight gain, obesity, high blood pressure and raised cholesterol levels. A diet high in added sugar from refined carbohydrates such as cakes and biscuits, as well as sweets and sugary drinks, can increase the likelihood of developing sight problems. Carbohydrates from processed and refined foods with little nutritional value are particularly bad for eyesight if eaten in quantity by picky eaters: a recent case in the news told of a seventeen-year-old teenager who had gone irreversibly blind after limiting his diet to only crisps, chips, white bread and processed meats since leaving primary school.[12] A similar outcome of blindness resulted for an eighteen-year-old who had eaten only a restricted diet of chocolate, crisps and chips since the age of two because he did not like the texture of other foods and refused to swallow them.[13] While these are extreme cases, whether a diet high in added sugar and refined carbohydrates will affect eyesight very much depends on the type of sugar eaten and how much.

FACT: _____

Many of the foods we buy contain more sugar than ever – pre-made food, especially – and it's making us unhealthy. Added sugar is even found in cans of tuna and many medicines, including those for children. High-sugar treats like fizzy drinks, sweets and fruits containing a lot of fructose such as mango and pineapple can increase the risk of developing eye diseases. Sugar also leaves the immune system less able to fight infection.

Persistently high blood glucose levels lead to insulin sensitivity – when the body's cells are unable to utilise insulin correctly due to too much glucose in the blood and/or too much fat around the cells. Even if a child or adult has not been diagnosed with pre-diabetes or Type 2 diabetes, mild symptoms can take years to be fully recognised. This is because the body tries to adapt to functioning with higher than normal blood glucose levels for a period of time by producing more and more insulin to deal with the excess glucose. However, these metabolic abnormalities begin to cause changes in the tiny blood vessels, first seen in the eyes and nerves. It may be years before sight loss is advanced enough to be noticeable, but the degenerative process is nonetheless present.

If blood glucose levels are higher than normal over a sustained period of time, i.e. not just on occasions such as a birthday party when a large amount of sugar has been consumed, these changes to the small blood vessels at the back of the eye can cause the condition known as retinopathy. Retinopathy causes the blood vessels in the retinas at the back of the eyes to leak and new blood vessels then grow abnormally. When the condition is mild it will make little difference to eyesight but the condition will progress if you consume a high-sugar diet over time causing sight to deteriorate. Retinopathy is one of the leading causes of sight loss and blindness in people with diabetes.

FACT: _____

Eating a reduced-sugar diet is the best way to prevent and manage retinopathy, allowing insulin to work properly to lower blood glucose levels.

Consuming a high-sugar diet can also increase the risk of developing the eye condition, macular degeneration. This is a condition usually associated with older age that causes loss of central vision, but consuming added sugar in large quantities accelerates the degeneration process, meaning macular degeneration can develop much earlier in life. Equally, high blood glucose levels can lead to cataracts. Cataracts describe clouding of the lens of the eye caused by protein deposits affecting central vision. High blood glucose levels increase swelling, fluid build-up and pressure in the eyes, allowing more protein to stick to the lens. Similarly, increased eye pressures can be caused by narrowing of the vessels supplying the eyes with blood, preventing the eyes from draining correctly. Elevated pressure in one or both eyes is worsened by a high-sugar diet and raised blood glucose levels. Increased eye pressure may eventually lead to the condition glaucoma.

TIP: _____

Choose healthier options with a lower sugar content to reduce blood glucose levels and the risk of developing any of the eye conditions mentioned above. If you are fighting sugar cravings and are tempted to break open the sweets or chocolate when sitting in front of the TV, consider that this decision may affect your long-term eye health.

Kidney problems

If blood glucose levels are higher than normal over time, this can damage the kidneys. Deposits of calcium collect within the kidneys to form kidney stones after only one year of eating a high-sugar diet. People who have kidney stones also have higher blood glucose levels, similar to those found in people with diabetes. High blood glucose levels passing through the kidneys over time destroy the structure of kidney tissue as glucose is a large molecule. Although the kidneys continue to function, this structural damage impairs the function. Consuming more sugar for as little as two weeks – over Christmas or on holiday, for example – can reduce the body's tolerance for glucose. A high-sugar diet increases fasting blood glucose levels – the amount of glucose in the blood before eating breakfast.

A reduced-sugar diet will protect the kidneys by slowing or preventing the formation of kidney stones and any structural damage to kidney tissue.

Tooth decay

In the UK, the level of tooth decay in children has fallen with the use of fluoride in toothpaste and regular dental checks, but the average child still has teeth that have been filled or that show some decay. One quarter of five-year-olds in England now has tooth decay. Tooth decay is a good indicator of whether your child's diet includes excessive amounts of sugar. Decay is caused by bacteria in the mouth that are stimulated by the consumption of sugar or starch. Sticky foods with a high-sugar content like sweets and biscuits cling to the teeth, leading to the breakdown of tooth enamel to cause decay. Damage to tooth enamel is caused by specific bacteria in the mouth, *streptococcus mutans*, that feed on a combination of glucose and fructose. As a result, sticky plaque is produced that clings to the surface of the teeth and around the gums while lactic acid, which is also in the plaque, gradually erodes the dentine surface to expose the soft pulp beneath. In the absence of fructose in the diet, any lactic acid produced is washed away by saliva, so there is no opportunity for tooth decay. This is the reason why fruit juice has been found to be particularly bad for children's teeth.

FACT: _____

In 1592, tooth decay was the fourth biggest killer after plague, fever and tuberculosis. The Tudors would sometimes 'clean' their teeth with sugar and honey because they knew no better. This had a similar effect on tooth decay as we see today in children and adults who do not brush their teeth regularly and thoroughly.

Dental problems are common in children and every year millions of teeth are extracted. One-third of adults in the UK over the age of sixteen have had a tooth extracted.[14] Tooth decay is this common because of sugar in the diet. A known cause of tooth decay is when children do not clean their teeth properly, made worse by consuming sweets, cakes, biscuits and soft drinks. Despite the knowledge that sugary foods and drinks cause tooth decay, children are still given them to eat, or children choose to buy them with pocket money. Tooth decay can be reduced with good dental hygiene and the reduction of a high starch and sugar diet that allows bacteria in the mouth to multiply.

Sam says, 'My seven-year-old son Kieran is notoriously bad at cleaning his teeth. Although we have tried to get him into a good routine and the dentist has shown him how to clean thoroughly, Kieran wasn't interested. I wanted to help him see why this was important so I looked up some websites on tooth decay with scary photographs. Kieran's attitude used to be that his milk teeth would be replaced, so it didn't matter if he cleaned them or not. The photos on the websites seem to have really worked and Kieran has said he doesn't want broken, black stumps in his mouth or his permanent teeth to be removed because of decay.'

We sometimes forget that as well as serious health implications like Type 2 diabetes, an excess of free sugars in the diet leads to plaque and bacteria build-up on teeth, causing more damage to them than any other food. Making the right food choices can have a big effect on the level of tooth decay that occurs. Here are some tips:

- Natural sugars in fruit and vegetables that are contained within the produce itself (as opposed to added) are far less likely than free sugars to cause tooth decay.

- Avoid eating dried fruits as a snack to reduce the damage done to teeth.

- Fruit juice or blended smoothies contain sugars that have been extracted from the produce, so these natural sugars become free sugars that can damage tooth enamel. While these foods appear healthy, it is advisable to drink only a small glass – 150ml of fruit juice or blended smoothies – per day to limit tooth decay.

- Drinks such as full-sugar juice drinks, fizzy drinks, soft drinks and fruit squashes are a major cause of tooth decay and should not be part of a child's diet.

- Always choose sugar-free fizzy drinks and squashes, milk or water for children to drink.

Finally, cleaning teeth after eating sweet foods is the ideal way of preventing tooth decay and this should be done whenever possible; it may even act as a deterrent to eating high-sugar foods if your child doesn't like brushing their teeth.

Gum problems leading to heart disease

As well as being a major cause of tooth decay, excess free sugar in the diet can also cause gum disease that affects the heart. You may think this is a strange relationship as the gums in the mouth are a long way from where the heart resides in the chest, but the condition of the teeth and gums affects overall health. Bacteria from decaying teeth can enter the bloodstream to affect the heart valves and kidneys.

FACT: _____
Gum disease increases a person's risk of heart disease by 20 per cent. Gum disease may increase heart disease risk because inflammation in the gums and bacteria can eventually lead to narrowing of coronary arteries.
_____

Gum disease is an infection of the tissues that support the teeth. This type of inflammation is usually due to bacteria from plaque build-up. Some people are more prone to gum disease because they have a weakened immune system, perhaps because they are very young, elderly or have a chronic health condition. Their bodies overreact to the plaque bacteria resulting in excessive inflammation around the gums. Often this does not get better quickly. When there is a high degree of bacteria present in the mouth, it can travel into the bloodstream, causing gradual damage to the blood vessels of the heart and brain over a number of years. Maintaining a healthy, low-sugar diet reduces the risk of gum disease and the risk of future damage to the blood vessels.

The main signs of gum disease in adults and children are:

- Bleeding gums when brushing or flossing.

- Gums that are red, swollen or tender.

- Gums that have pulled away from the teeth.

- Ongoing bad breath.

- Loose teeth.

Coronary thrombosis: the modern epidemic

Coronary thrombosis is the formation of a blood clot inside a blood vessel of the heart. A diet high in sugars encourages abdominal fat to accumulate in the cells and this is a significant risk factor for the development of heart disease compared to fat deposits elsewhere in the body, such as in the legs. It is now clear that the causes of heart disease are more complicated than just eating a high-fat diet. Other risk factors include increased blood pressure, hormonal disturbances, changes in the way that blood clots, an increased level of blood glucose and an associated rise in the level of insulin present in the blood. A high-sugar diet promotes each of these risk factors. High blood glucose levels and increased insulin to reduce glucose levels are also associated with fatty deposits in the arteries, encouraging blood clot formation. Coronary heart disease and Type 2 diabetes are inextricably linked to a diet that contains sugar.

FACT: _____

In the UK, there are 7.4 million people currently living with heart and circulatory problems.

Cholesterol describes fatty deposits in the blood, the level of which increases as we get older. Some of this cholesterol sticks to the artery walls – known as atherosclerosis – especially the arteries that supply blood to the heart for pumping around the body. As these arteries narrow because of cholesterol deposits, less blood is able to reach the heart and this causes a condition called angina pectoris where there is pain in the chest when exercise is taken. The presence of cholesterol on the artery walls also increases the likelihood of blood clot formation which can lead to a blockage in one of the arteries that supplies the heart with blood. This restricts blood flow to an area of the heart, leading to a heart attack.

FACT: _____

Atherosclerosis – the narrowing of the arteries – can occur in any artery in the body and is known to start as early as the teenage years, while some studies suggest even earlier. As it develops, it may cause pain in the legs (peripheral vascular disease) or chest (angina) when exercising.

Coronary heart disease

A restriction of blood to the heart – coronary artery disease – manifests as a rise in blood fats such as low-density lipids (LDL), cholesterol and triglycerides. There is also an increase in blood glucose levels in adults and children without diabetes and an associated rise in the amount of insulin found in the blood, a rise in the uric acid level – the cause of gout – and a change in blood platelets so that they clot more readily. The consumption of a high-sugar diet is harmful to younger people and this group is more likely to eat a diet containing a greater quantity of soft drinks, ice cream, cakes and biscuits than older people. Research has shown that 25–30 per cent of the population has an increased sensitivity to dietary sugar in the body, such as the formation of atherosclerosis in the arteries.

Links with certain cancers

A study in the British Medical Journal examining 100,000 people over five years stated that consuming sugary drinks increases the risk of developing certain cancers.[15] In the UK, one can of sugary drink is 330ml and, according to the study, drinking 100ml more than this per day increases the risk of developing cancer by 18 per cent. The study showed that the average person consumed two cans of sugary drink per day. Drinking four cans of sugary drink per day increased the risk by 32 per cent. While both adults and children enjoy eating and drinking sweet treats because they are comforting and satisfy cravings, the unpleasant truth is that a diet high in foods containing free sugars – cakes, biscuits, sweets, chocolate, fizzy drinks, syrups and smoothies – increases the risk of developing certain cancers as well as obesity, heart disease and Type 2 diabetes.

Cancers of the pancreas, breast and large intestine are diagnosed more frequently among individuals who eat a diet high in refined, high-sugar, high-calorie foods than in those who eat a healthy, low-sugar diet, rich in natural grains with no added sugars.[16,17,18] The key to identifying these foods is to study food labels. Make sure you cut out additional sugars in drinks, baking and cereal in your own and your child's diet. As we have already seen, sugar is added to foods during the manufacturing process to make it taste nice. This applies to savoury foods that you might not expect to contain a high amount of added sugar, such as soups, sauces, pickled onions, tinned meats and some brands of tuna fish.

FACT: _____

The UK has one of the highest rates of breast cancer in the world and also a higher rate of sugar consumption when compared with other countries.

The development of breast cancer has been shown to be related to hormonal levels in the body. Sugar is responsible for disrupting the levels of several hormones, so a reduction of sugar intake can reduce the chances of developing breast cancer. It has also been shown that high blood insulin levels caused by eating a high-sugar diet can lead to cancer of the large intestine.[19] A link has also been found between the development of testicular cancer in young men when their mother was overweight with an increased level of oestrogen in their bloodstream.[20] A diet that is high in sugar results in a high concentration of insulin and oestrogen in the blood.

FACT: _____

It is often claimed that children now reach puberty earlier than they did a century ago due to a more nutritious diet. Research has shown that children become sexually mature at an earlier age if they eat a high-sugar diet because sugar has an effect on hormone levels.[21]

Reduced immune system function

The immune system fights disease when we get an infection such as a cold or flu. The immune system works less efficiently when there is a high amount of sugar present in the diet or when diabetes is not controlled properly. Bacteria and yeast feed on sugar, which means an infection could be prolonged and can encourage further infection, challenging an already weakened immune system.

Affluent countries such as the UK tend to produce well-nourished children compared to less wealthy countries, though research shows that this can stray into overindulgence with babies in the UK now frequently overweight. Bottle-fed babies tend to weigh more than babies who are breast-fed and as a result, overweight children tend to reach maturity quicker and tend to be taller than their normal-weight counterparts. Bottled milk formula contains added sugar, encouraging an early reliance on sweet foods, whereas breast milk contains milk sugar, which is still sugar but not as sweet nor artificial. Bottle-fed babies often experience diarrhoea and vomiting as a result of consuming milk containing sucrose when compared with breast-fed babies who are only getting lactose, and who also receive immunity from breast milk against harmful bacteria.

FACT: _____

Eating sugar or foods containing sugar can make adults and children feel unwell, lethargic, quick to become tired, achy and prone to periodic infections.

Indigestion and gallstones

People who are under a lot of stress often suffer from severe indigestion. Even this can be significantly improved in many cases with a low-sugar, low-carbohydrate diet. Sugar promotes the production of excess stomach acid and the stomach lining becomes far more sensitive. A diet with less sugar can help alleviate these symptoms.

Shirley says, 'I was diagnosed with gallstones and high cholesterol levels in my late teens after visiting my doctor with a constant pain in my right side. Because I was overweight, my risk of developing Type 2 diabetes was increased. Several members of my family already had this condition. I was advised to eat a low-fat diet but that only helped with the pain a small amount. I found an article online about cholesterol being linked to sugar in the diet so I started cutting it out of tea and coffee and stopped sugary snacks, which I didn't really miss after a few weeks. My doctor carried out a second ultrasound examination six months later to check the status of the gallstones and they hadn't got any bigger. My weight had also decreased and I was told I'd significantly improved my chances of not developing Type 2 diabetes.'

A steady intake of added sugars and refined carbohydrates can increase the risk of developing gallstones because more insulin is needed to metabolise these foods. Elevated insulin levels increase the concentration of cholesterol in the bile. Gallstones are solid particles in the gallbladder that are formed of bile cholesterol and are increasingly being diagnosed in younger individuals. When gallstones are diagnosed, additional health issues are usually also discovered. These include obesity, Type 2 diabetes and high levels of insulin and blood fats – cholesterol and triglycerides. Reducing sugar in the diet slows down or prevents cholesterol from forming into gallstones.

Skin conditions caused or made worse by sugar

Some skin conditions have been linked to the consumption of sugar in the diet, most notably a condition known as seborrheic dermatitis, where the glands secrete the oily substance sebum, the structure of which is altered when a high-sugar diet is consumed. As with all the health conditions discussed in this book, a low-sugar diet improves this skin condition.

Liz says, 'My daughter, Kierra, developed terrible acne in her early teens that the family doctor put down to adolescence. The condition had such an impact on Kierra that she wouldn't go out and she would always pull her hair over her face so people couldn't see the red, angry skin. I asked the doctor to refer us to a dermatologist who recommended creams and antibiotic treatment. She also suggested improving Kierra's diet by cutting sugary drinks and sweets because the bacteria causing the acne responded to the sugar, making the condition worse. We did everything we were told to do and after a couple of months, there was a real improvement with Kierra's skin looking less red and the spots beginning to heal.'

You may wonder why I have included some 'adult' diseases in this chapter, but this is to emphasise the dangers of a high-sugar diet and the importance of preventing your child from developing these illnesses in the future. A key issue concerning a high-sugar diet from birth onwards is the effect dietary sugar has on the body's ability to use protein. Protein forms the building blocks of the body but it is disrupted by the presence of sugar, rendering it less effective so that it breaks down and is excreted before it can encourage growth. This can be measured by the amount of nitrogen present in the urine as the body removes the by-products of protein metabolism; a diet high in sugar will cause a greater amount of nitrogen to be excreted in the urine, indicating that protein is being lost, when compared with a diet that is low in sugar.

KEY MESSAGES IN THIS CHAPTER

- A high-sugar diet affects every bodily system because blood glucose reaches every part of the body.

- A high-sugar diet is associated with a range of health issues including obesity, Type 2 diabetes, heart disease and certain cancers. These health problems are now being seen in young people and some children.

- Compared to an adult, a child is far more sensitive to a sudden rise or fall in blood glucose.

- Natural sugars in fruit and vegetables contained within the produce itself are far less likely than free sugars to cause tooth decay.

- Always choose sugar-free fizzy drinks and squashes, milk or water for children to drink.

Alternatives to Sugar

We have now seen how sugar can affect the body in many different ways if eaten to excess over a period of time. This may make you want to avoid sugar as far as possible in the family diet but this brings with it concerns, such as how to make food taste good when sugar is removed or reduced, and whether the family will enjoy mealtimes less as a result. The following chapter looks at the difference between alternative sugars and artificial sweeteners, the numerous alternatives to sugar that are available and how they can be used in a healthier diet. I also discuss how sugar alternatives and sweeteners are made and the products that contain them to enable you to make an informed decision about including alternatives to sugar in your family's diet or not.

The difference between alternative sugars and artificial sweeteners

Alternative sugars are derived from natural sources such as raisin sugar, agave syrup and honey, and are used to sweeten foods. Alternative sugars added to foods by manufacturers are dextrose, glucose, glucose syrup, lactose, maltose, maltodextrin and maltodextrose. These sugars are derived from substances like milk to sweeten baby formulas and from glucose, which is a simple sugar that our bodies use for energy.

Artificial sweeteners are either derived from sugar or are created chemically using sugars that are absorbed by the body in a different way to sucrose and glucose. Sugar substitutes are produced by altering the structure of the sugar molecule to make it into a substance called sorbitol. Depending on the chemical alteration, different artificial sweeteners can be produced, such as maltitol and xylitol, although they are not as sweet as sugar. These artificial sweeteners also cause diarrhoea, so only small amounts can be eaten safely.

TIP:
Because sugar substitutes are sweeter than sugar, less is needed to enhance the flavour of food with the advantage that fewer calories are consumed; this is useful in a calorie-controlled diet.

Fructose and high-fructose corn syrup
Many foods are now sweetened with fructose or high-fructose corn syrup. Fruit sugar has been in the human diet for millennia so our digestive systems are used to small quantities. But we don't just eat a handful of berries in their natural form picked from a bush or a couple of apples a day, quantities that our bodies can deal with. We now consume fruit juice that is concentrated with fruit sugar minus the fibre of the original fruit. This means that much of the fruit we now eat is processed – pie filling, jam, fruit juices, fruit snacks, smoothies and fruit desserts. We believe that eating fruit in any form is good because it's one of our five-a-day, but this is not the case.

FACT:
Without the fibre from fruit skins, anything over 10g of consumed fruit sugar can cause damage in the body. Make sure you eat fruit in its natural form.

Pria says, 'I always used to think that seeing "no added sugar" on a product I bought for my kids was a good thing but then I discovered that these foods are sweetened with fruit sugar – fruit sugar is still sugar. It can be difficult to find healthy alternatives to family favourites so I make as many things as I can at home to reduce the sugar content. I know this isn't for everyone, but it's a good way of reducing sugar. You can also check labels and compare similar products to see which ones are made with less sugar. The thing is to be aware of naturally sweetened foods, especially products sweetened with fructose syrup, and don't assume they're healthy.'

Alternatively, sweetened foods should only be consumed short term if you are trying to reduce your family's sugar intake. Consuming foods containing sugar substitutes doesn't allow a sugar dependency to be overcome because they taste sweet, perpetuating cravings for sugar. Some sweeteners – like sorbitol which can cause diarrhoea – should not be consumed at all if possible, especially not by children in several daily fizzy drinks or sugar-free sweets, while other sweeteners are safe to consume in small quantities.

You may want to decide based on the information given in this book which alternative sweeteners you and your family will eat and those you'd rather avoid, based on potential adverse effects such as diarrhoea and the taste of the product. Sometimes it's difficult to assess how a food like yoghurt has been sweetened, although you assume it's with natural lactose sugars rather than an alternative sweetener. Manufacturers are permitted to use additives in food, which are listed as E-numbers to show alternative sweeteners and colours in the product ingredients. Unless you can decipher these numbers, you may be buying something with a sweetener you'd rather not eat.

Should I include alternative sweeteners in my family's diet?

Alternative sweeteners which offer a high intensity of sweetness when compared with sugar are listed on manufacturer's labels with the following E-numbers:

E950 = Acesulphame potassium

E956 = Alitame

E951 = Aspartame

E962 = Aspartame-acesuphame

E952 = Cyclamates

E968 = Erythritol

E961= Neotame

E954 = Saccharin

E960 = Stevia

E955 = Sucralose

E967 = Xylitol

The advantages and disadvantages of available alternative sweeteners are shown below:

- ACESULFAME POTASSIUM (E950) is widely used to sweeten many foods and is often mixed with other sweeteners, especially aspartame, by food manufacturers to reduce the artificial taste.

- ALITAME (E956) is 2,000 times sweeter than sugar and ten times as sweet as aspartame, so only a very small amount is added to foods by manufacturers. It cannot be used in foods that have to be heated as alitame breaks down when cooked, but its advantage is that it's not broken down into phenylalanine by the body so it is safe for people with the condition phenylketonuria. Alitame is not permitted in the United States or the UK but it is used in Australia, New Zealand and China.

- ASPARTAME (E951) is not a low-calorie sweetener like saccharin and cyclamate; aspartame has equal calories to sugar but is 200 times sweeter so less is eaten to achieve the same sweetness. Aspartame – sold as NutraSweet and Equal – is formed partly from methyl alcohol that's digested by the body and broken down by the liver into formaldehyde. A

2014 mega-study[1] examining the dangers of aspartame by collecting results from a number of other studies showed that aspartame was a 'moderate genotoxic agent' with a 73 per cent positive result across all studies for cancers of the brain, prostate, breast, lymph glands, blood, kidneys and ureters, skin and nerves. Despite this, aspartame sweetener is available in the United States as NutraSweet and Equal, while the World Health Organisation declared aspartame safe in 1974. Diet Pepsi stopped using this sweetener because of ongoing consumer concern. In the US, the maximum daily limit of aspartame is 50mg per kg of bodyweight per day, while in Europe, the recommended amount is 40mg/kg/day.

FACT: _____

Children with the medical condition phenylketonuria – an intolerance to phenylalanine amino acid found in most proteins – should not be given food and drinks sweetened with aspartame.

- CYCLAMATE (E952) is fifty times sweeter than sugar and passes through the body undigested, so it is used as a low-calorie sweetener. On its own it has an unpleasant taste like saccharin, although when saccharin and cyclamate are combined to sweeten food and drink the effect is reduced and only a small amount is needed to achieve the sweetness of sugar. This combination of cyclamate and saccharin was used commercially as a product called Sweet'N Low. Cyclamate is still used in products in the UK but has been banned in the US since 1969 because research showed it increased the risk of developing cancer and also caused testicular degeneration, reducing sperm production.

- NEOTAME (E961) is 13,000 times sweeter than sugar and, like aspartame and alitame, is derived from aspartic acid found in plant proteins. Similar to alitame, neotame cannot be used to sweeten foods that will be heated because it will break down. However, because it is sourced from plant proteins, neotame is not broken down into phenylalanine during digestion. Neotame has a wider use than alitame as it is permitted in foods in the UK, the United States, Australia and New Zealand.

- SACCHARIN (E954) is probably the best-known artificial sweetener, with other low-calorie sugar substitutes now available such as aspartame. However, these sweeteners do not have the same ability as sugar to add bulk to foods and they cannot be used as a preserving agent in the same way, as sugar prevents microbes growing and contaminating food. For these reasons, saccharin and aspartame are only used to sweeten beverages like manufactured drinks and tea and coffee.

   Saccharin is 300 times sweeter than sugar and has been used for more than 140 years as a sugar alternative and a low-calorie alternative as it passes through the body undigested. It is sold as the product Sugar Twin but it leaves an unpalatable metallic taste in the mouth. It has been used to sweeten products for people with diabetes. Personally, I avoid it, preferring to go without the taste of 'metal jam'. Although table top saccharin to sweeten tea and coffee is still allowed, it has been delisted for use as a food additive in Canada because it was found to cause cancer in rats but was later found to have no effect on humans. Saccharin is still available as an alternative sweetener in the UK.

FACT: _____

Both saccharin and aspartame sweeteners cannot be heated in cooking as their compounds become unstable.

- STEVIA – E960 – is a plant-based derivative that is up to 400 times sweeter than sugar depending on which part of the plant is used. It combines glucose and steviol. This alternative sweetener is not permitted in the United States due to concerns that it has contributed to the onset of Type 2 diabetes because it does contain glucose. Only a small amount is required to sweeten foods and drinks, and stevia is permitted in the UK as it's not considered to be harmful in minute quantities.

- SUCRALOSE (E955) is 600 times sweeter than sugar and is sold as the alternative sweetener Splenda, which is permitted in the UK. It is not a low-calorie sweetener but less is needed to achieve a sweet taste in food, so fewer calories are consumed. Sucralose is used by the soft drinks industry and, unlike other sweeteners, can be used in cooking because it maintains its structure when heated. Sucralose also looks like sugar, being granulated.

FACT: _____

Alternative sweeteners should not be used as a replacement for sugar over the long term if you are trying to drastically reduce or remove sugar from your diet as sweeteners do not enable you to overcome a sugar dependency.

Consume with caution!

The alternative sweetener sorbitol can have adverse effects on the digestive system if eaten in quantity, causing diarrhoea and stomach pains in adults and children. Foods for people with diabetes are sweetened with sorbitol, as are 'low-sugar' cough syrups and some other medications for children. Around 15 per cent of the sorbitol used to sweeten foods passes into the large intestine where it takes in water to cause unpleasant symptoms. There are other alternative sweeteners listed below that should be consumed with caution because they are combined with a great deal of fructose; they are metabolised into fructose during digestion; or they are high-sugar alternatives that won't help achieve either weight loss or a low-sugar lifestyle:

Agave syrup; corn syrup; fructose; fruit juice concentrate; golden syrup; high-fructose corn syrup; honey; inulin; E953 Isomalt; E966 Lactitol; litesse; E965 Maltitol; E421 Mannitol; maple syrup; molasses; polydextrose; resistant dextrin; E420 Sorbitol; sucrose; wheat dextrin.

There are further substances known as sugar alcohols which pass through the body unchanged but can cause digestive disturbance if eaten in large quantities:

- ERYTHRITOL (E968) glucose is extracted from fermented corn or wheat starch. It is a very low-calorie sugar alcohol and the majority of its structure passes through the body undigested.

- ISOMALT (E953) is a sugar alcohol formed from glucose, sorbitol and mannitol. Sorbitol and mannitol are converted into fructose during digestion. Isomalt does not increase blood glucose levels or trigger the release of insulin.

- LACTITOL (E956) is manufactured from lactose and has been used since the 1980s. The human digestive system does not absorb lactitol sugar alcohol so it passes directly into the large intestine where it releases fatty acids into the bloodstream.

- MALTITOL (E965) is a sugar alcohol with a similar sweetness to sugar. It is broken down into sorbitol and glucose and converted into fructose. Maltitol has 75–90 per cent of the sweetness of sugar and looks very similar, although it can cause diarrhoea.

- MANNITOL (E421) is a sugar alcohol made from hydrogen and fructose and is treated by the body like fructose during digestion.

- POLYDEXTROSE (E1200) is manufactured from glucose and sorbitol and is a glucan – a substance known as a polysaccharide. Polydextrose adds consistency and volume to food but does not add sweetness. Polydextrose is used to treat constipation because it is a plant fibre, and pre-diabetes and Type 2 diabetes because the fibre acts to reduce blood glucose levels. In foods, polydextrose is used as a sweetener and to improve the texture of foods, adding bulk to diet and low-sugar foods. Although polydextrose is not sweet it contains many molecules of glucose, breaking down into glucose.

- SORBITOL (E420) is a sugar alcohol that is marketed as a laxative because it draws water into the large intestine. It is also used as an alternative sweetener for diabetic foods, low-sugar cough syrups and children's allergy medicines such as Piriton syrup. Because of sorbitol's effect on the large intestine, it is not suitable for people with irritable bowel syndrome. Sorbitol becomes fructose when it is broken down by the body, which is quickly converted into stored glucose (glycogen and triglycerides) by the liver.

- XYLITOL (E967) is a sugar alcohol used as an alternative sweetener because only two-thirds of its calorie content can be absorbed by the human digestive system. Xylitol is extracted from birch wood and has been found to be beneficial in reducing tooth decay when used in chewing gum and mouthwash.

Some alternative sugars are not food additives. These are made from natural fibre and pass through the body without being absorbed:

- INULIN is a natural alternative to sugar that is made from a chain of sugar molecules and is common in many plants, where it is used to store energy. Inulin can be found in the coffee substitute chicory. Inulin is digested as fibre, which the human body can't process for energy like other carbohydrates so it passes into the small intestine. Like other dietary fibres, inulin may promote gut health and helps to manage blood glucose levels.

- WHEAT DEXTRIN is a chemically altered soluble wheat starch that is widely used to add bulk to processed foods. Wheat dextrin has been marketed as a cholesterol-lowering substance but it has downsides: wheat dextrin can stimulate the pancreas to release insulin and disrupt the storage of glucose as glycogen in the liver, thus interfering with blood glucose levels.

In summary, inulin, polydextrose and wheat dextrin are fibrous substances that cannot be digested because humans do not have the correct enzymes to do this. Intestinal bacteria feed on the sugars in these high-fibre foods and convert them into fatty acids.

Are artificial sweeteners safe?

Although alternative sweeteners are used widely by the food industry, some of the chemical compounds manufactured to replicate sugar, such as aspartame and cyclamate, have been shown to increase the risk of developing cancer. With this knowledge, you can now make an informed choice regarding whether to include these sweeteners in your family's diet or not. If you include them, it does not mean that cancer is inevitable: these chemicals have only been shown to increase the risk of developing cancer rather than definitely causing it. In addition, studies showing the development of cancer in rats fed on alternative sweeteners have been accelerated to mimic the likely disease path seen in humans over a lifetime, using much larger amounts of sweetener than a human may ever consume.

Foods that contain alternative sweeteners should only be consumed in the short term if you want to overcome sugar dependence in the long term. Some sweeteners, like aspartame, should not be consumed at all if possible because methyl alcohol is used in its manufacture. Studies have shown that this substance is a moderate genotoxic agent. While seemingly safe amounts of methyl alcohol are permitted in fizzy drinks, children's bodies are far smaller than an adult and are more sensitive to the effects of chemicals. Any substance that is broken down into formaldehyde will change the structure of body cells because it affects the protein within them.

KEY MESSAGES IN THIS CHAPTER

- Alternative sweeteners are either derived from sugar or are created chemically using sugars that are absorbed by the body in a different way to sucrose and glucose.
- Foods that contain alternative sweeteners instead of sugar should only be consumed in the short term if you are trying to reduce your family's sugar intake.
- Children with the medical condition phenylketonuria – an intolerance to the phenylalanine amino acid found in most proteins – should not be given food and drinks sweetened with aspartame.
- Although alternative sweeteners are used widely by the food industry, some of the chemical compounds manufactured to replicate sugar have been shown to be unsafe if consumed regularly and in large quantities, such as in fizzy drinks or foods sweetened with aspartame or sorbitol. With this knowledge, you can make an informed choice about whether to include foods and drinks sweetened with chemical alternatives to sugar in your family's diet.

Breaking the Habit

There is no doubt that sugar is a highly addictive substance that has little nutritional value, as well as causing or exacerbating a number of health problems. In this chapter, I will show you how to break a sugar addiction in stages rather than going 'cold turkey' and stopping all sugars in one go. When tackling a sugar dependency, it is more effective to cut down gradually on sugar in stages, meal by meal, so that new patterns of behaviour become permanent lifestyle changes. Making dietary changes will be much harder to do if you try to do lots of different things in one go, and this will increase the likelihood of giving up on the idea that sugar can be reduced as much as possible from the family diet.

Why sugar is so addictive

Dopamine is a chemical transmitter produced in several areas of the brain that provides a feeling of well-being. The brain releases dopamine to support behaviours that are important for survival, such as eating food. Sugar helps us to absorb the amino acid tryptophan, which is used to make the neurotransmitter serotonin. The interaction of sugar with the pleasure centres of the brain causes the release of more dopamine and this is why we perceive eating sugary foods and drinks as comforting, but this only lasts for a short time so we crave more sugar to get the same effect. If we do something that creates a dopamine release again and again, such as having sugary snacks between meals to boost our mood, we become addicted. Addictive substances like heroin, nicotine and sugar increase the dopamine response in the body and because dopamine promotes memory, understanding, motivation and reward, we remember feeling good and want to repeat the activity that created that feeling again.

FACT: _____

It takes three weeks to break a bad habit such as eating a daily bar of chocolate. Forming a new habit, like taking some exercise every day, takes three months to establish.

It is possible to tackle an addiction to sugar in the same way as any addiction. A good way to start reducing sugar intake is to cut down in stages rather than cutting sugar out of your life suddenly and completely. By reducing sugar week by week, this makes the process much easier to manage. It helps to have an incentive for cutting down – improving general health or preventing tooth decay so that your child's dentist can say that no new fillings are necessary, for example. Reduce the amount of sugar added to drinks and cereal as a start, then continue with confectionery, cakes and biscuits in the diet. Buy diet soft drinks instead of full-sugar varieties that are alternatively sweetened in a way you're happy with. You can also reduce the amount of sugary desserts your child eats, and save them as a special treat rather than as a regular end to a meal. Replace sugary cereals with healthier varieties such as Shredded Wheat, Weetabix or porridge oats.

FACT: _____

When sugar is reduced in the diet the taste buds are better able to distinguish differences in the flavour, meaning you are able to enjoy food more. The way we assess how sweet our food and drink tastes is not only a subjective process: sweetness is affected by factors such as the acidity level of the food or drink; its temperature; and, in the case of drinks like orange squash, how much it's diluted with water.

Look at food packaging to find the sugars contained in the bread or cereal your child is eating. The packaging might say '15g of sugar per serving', but has your child been eating the same quantity as the manufacturer's serving suggestion? Perhaps your child has been consuming closer to two or three servings in weight. To make your child more aware of what they are eating you could measure out grams of sugar to see what this amount really looks like. A teaspoon of sugar is 4g, so a portion of cereal containing 20g of sugar is equal to your child eating five teaspoons of sugar. When sugar is weighed out and seen as a physical entity in front of them, children are amazed that they are eating so much sugar in their food because this makes it real. Children tend to ask for healthier options after you have done this exercise.

A similar exercise that helps children visualise the sugar content in non-diet fizzy drinks can be very effective too. It is based on something I was told by a nurse when I first developed Type 1 diabetes as a child, and it has stayed with me ever since. Explain to your child that there are eight teaspoons of sugar in a can of fizzy drink. All that sugar going into a little person from a can of fizzy drink is going to have a far greater effect on their mood and blood glucose levels than the same amount going into a teenager or an adult. You can show this by putting eight teaspoons of sugar into a small cup, then a large mug, then a jug and diluting it with water. If they take a small sip of the liquid from each container they can taste the result for themselves – the small cup of sugar water tastes really sweet compared with the jug of sugar water.

Liz says, 'My teenage son loves sugary cereal and he eats it as a snack as well as in the mornings. I've been worried about how much sugar he eats for some time but didn't know how to tackle the issue without it looking like nagging. After school one day I made a detour to the supermarket with my son and casually mentioned that I wanted to find a healthy cereal for my own breakfast. I don't generally eat cereal but thought he might follow by example. We stood in the breakfast foods aisle while I checked the nutrition information on a couple of boxes, mentioning that they all seemed high in sugar. My son then became interested and helped me look. He picked up a box of his own preferred cereal and read this information, seemed surprised at how high the sugar content was and he made a healthier choice with far less sugar. This has really made a difference and my son has said he now realises how sweet his preferred cereal was. This method of looking for something for yourself in the shops is a game that youngsters like to get involved in; it gets them looking at labels and thinking about the sugar in what they eat.'

The stages of change

At the very beginning as you embark on a low-sugar diet, instead of trying to change the world in one go or urging the whole family to go 'cold turkey' on high-sugar foods, just make very small changes gradually that will add up and make a huge difference. Children look to their parents for guidance, so if they see Mum and Dad eating porridge for breakfast rather than Crunchy Nut Cornflakes or Sugar Puffs, they will be more likely to want to copy and join in too. This also works the other way: when children see a parent behaving in a certain way because they have eaten or drunk something that affects their mood, they notice and even if they don't say anything at the time, they remember this effect. Studies have shown similar effects when children see their parents drinking alcohol and they learn the connection between alcohol and a change in behaviour.

FACT: _____

When a child reduces their sugar intake their behaviour is likely to change due to stabilised blood glucose levels and improved nutrition. The change is more noticeable than in an adult because children are more sensitive to the additives, chemicals and sugars in food and soft drinks.

Children love to discover new things and are naturally curious, as per Liz's example earlier, where her son chose a new cereal with a lower sugar content compared to his usual variety. During trips to the supermarket with your child, look at cereals or breakfast foods to choose one together that's lower in sugar. Depending on the age of the child, they may make their own decision to change how they eat after studying the labels. This is preferable to them being told to do something they don't want to do. Once a child discovers that they feel different because they've eaten something nutritious instead of a sugar-laden snack that makes them hyper then depressed and tired an hour or so later, they will want to repeat the good feelings and reduce or avoid the bad.

FACT:

Replacing high-sugar foods with those rich in protein and good carbohydrates means that mood swings, temper tantrums, poor concentration and erratic blood glucose levels are eliminated.

Helping your child to overcome the addiction

Reducing your child's sugar intake is about eating sensibly, not removing sugar completely from the diet as this is practically impossible. Enjoying something sweet occasionally will not lead to any disastrous consequences. It would be very difficult to do this with today's processed foods; the only way to avoid sugar completely would be to grow and prepare all your family's food yourself. Almost everything you can buy seems to have some variety of sugar added these days as a flavour enhancer, bulking agent or preservative, so choose foods labelled 'no added sugar' whenever possible.

TIP:

Make a list of sugary foods eaten over one week and make a game of reducing these foods the week after.

Recognise where habits might have formed in association with sweet foods as this is the first step towards breaking the sugar habit. Eating sugary foods can be part of a pleasurable event without us even realising it. Do you tend to visit the supermarket café when you go shopping as a family and enjoy having a sweet treat? Could you avoid the confectionary aisle? Do you always stop off at McDonalds as a reward after taking your child to the dentist for a check-up? Does your family tend to buy popcorn at the cinema and a large sugary drink to go with it? Could you and your children easily go without sweets or chocolate in the evening while watching TV? Help your child make a list of habits associated with food so you can all identify what's happening. It isn't always obvious when sugary snacks and foods are being eaten in addition to your usual meals.

Learn to recognise that the association of enjoyment is because of the activity – being with family and friends, seeing a film at the cinema, watching TV – rather than the sugary snacks themselves and this will help break the habit. Make healthier substitutions for these sugary snacks like eating unsalted nuts or reduced-fat potato or vegetable crisps in front of the TV, or taking your own unsweetened popcorn to the cinema with you. It can be fun to make popcorn at home and it's a healthy snack that's full of fibre. Discover what your food-associated habits are and make substitutions like seeing a film as a reward for an all-clear check-up at the dentist.

TIP:

Always eat a breakfast that includes protein and complex carbohydrates and eat it within an hour of waking to raise blood glucose levels that have dropped during sleep.

If you know that certain situations are associated with sugary snacks, try to change them if you can. If a visit to Grandma always involves her making a cake, explain to her that the family is trying to eat less sugar to be healthier. Grandma wants her family to be healthy, so she will support you.

Talk about acceptable alternatives rather than going without so no one feels deprived. You could write a list of ways to avoid sugar in social situations so you are prepared; for example, taking your own savoury, healthier snacks to the cinema rather than hoping to find something acceptable to eat once there when you are rushed for time. This could mean coming to an agreement with your child that you'll buy Shredded Wheat the next time you visit the supermarket instead of Sugar Puffs. Don't assume you or your child will be able to manage without sugar completely – it isn't going to be an automatic process like turning off a switch. Another example is if you are attending a children's party and there's a tableful of sweet things on offer – ensure you have strategies already in place and bring some acceptable choices with you. You will be able to find healthier savoury or 'no added sugar' alternatives that the party host will be happy with.

FACT: _____

Once sugar avoidance strategies are embedded in behaviour, the need for sugar – the addiction – will have gone.

Your own behaviour is the most influential factor on your child so if you are rushing around, grabbing a snack with little time to eat properly, they will take that on board. You need to do the same thing you are asking them to do: eat proper meals, don't leave it more than three hours between meals without eating something that isn't junk food, and so on. To reverse an old saying, 'Do as I do, not as I say.' Map out a plan, make small changes and take it slowly. By joining in, children begin to understand why lowering the amount of sugar they eat is really important so that it's not just seen as 'one of Mum or Dad's weird ideas'. Forced change does not have the desired effect on behaviour as a person must want to make a change and understand why they want things to be different. It is crucial that you make the changes with your children.

Reducing sugar in your child's diet
While it's difficult to know what your child might be eating when they are out with their friends or staying at their houses, as long as you reduce your child's sugar intake at home, this will mean they are eating far less sugar in the long run. Help your child understand how

certain foods can make them feel a certain way by keeping a food diary and add any feelings to the notes made. If you do ask questions when your child is writing their food diary, don't judge and don't bombard them. Show an interest and ask a few questions like, 'Do you look forward to eating breakfast in the morning because you're hungry?' or, 'What's your favourite thing for breakfast?' The answer to this last question may change if your child has recently switched from a high-sugar cereal to porridge, Weetabix or Shredded Wheat because they are no longer getting a quantity of sugar first thing.

If having sweets at a friend's house made your child feel happy then grumpy later, ask them to write that down so that they start to notice these associations. In this way over time, these connections will become learned behaviour and your child will be more aware of what happens when they eat and drink different foods. You could also do this and the fact that Mum or Dad are joining in will be encouraging. You can show them what's in your own food diary and they will be able to understand how you felt after eating certain foods too. You might even find them giving you advice like, 'You know that cake with the coffee icing gives you a sugar rush, so don't buy any!'

When you are first planning to reduce the amount of sugar, just write down what is eaten and when, how much and what effect it had. Don't start cutting certain foods out of the family diet straight away. Begin by finding out the information you need to show exactly what your family is eating. Find out what your children eat in and out of the home and when. If your children are older, let them have a notebook of their own so they can write down what they eat and feel involved in the process. Don't make any comments about what they write because then they won't share the details and try not to be insistent – just find out in an easy-going way what your children eat and when.

FACT: _____

The ability to make an informed choice is based on the information available to you and your child.

Sally says, 'When I've dieted in the past, I wrote down the calories in everything I ate. I adapted this method for sugar and suggested the whole family did the same so we could be healthier. We started in the school holidays; it was difficult to remember at first and both my children had their own notebooks, but when I wrote down what I'd eaten, they did the same. This became a habit after a while and it was easy to see where we were going wrong with sweet treats. I then asked them to write down how they felt and I did the same. We soon discovered that feeling happier after eating sugar was short-lived, followed by feeling fed-up, tired and grouchy. Once we could see how sweet stuff affected us, it was easier to cut it out and have healthier, filling foods instead, like porridge or Shredded Wheat for breakfast instead of Coco Pops.'

We have all witnessed the exasperated parent in the supermarket who is stressed and annoyed by their child's behaviour. If your child is struggling to behave while out in public, treat the cause of the problem rather than asking your child, 'Why are you acting in this way?' Give them a banana to increase their glucose levels. It's impossible for you or your child to make rational associations between food and behaviour if their blood glucose levels are low.

Encourage the family to write down what they eat and how they feel. This can really help to show how eating certain foods affects moods and emotions. As well as your food diary, you may want to keep a written record of which snacks and fizzy drinks disappear from the kitchen over the course of one week as a way of keeping track of the types of food your child eats. If you have more than one child, they may each have different preferences.

You could then look at your supermarket and fast-food till receipts so you can see what you're spending on certain snack foods. See what kinds of carbohydrates, proteins, fruit and vegetables feature on these receipts and involve your child in the process as a game, noting any differences between individual food preferences.

Be aware of what you are buying and what your family is eating as the information you gather will allow you to see where change is needed. When you ask your child what they are eating at school or at a friend's house you can only trust they are telling the truth. They may think they'll get in trouble if you find out they ate crisps and Coke for lunch, so be an impartial observer and don't make a big deal out of the question or their answers.

As well as looking at receipts for information, you could make a game of discovering how much protein and carbohydrate your child has each day by looking up the values online of what they have entered into their food diary. If they become involved in this way, they will want to work out what they are having over a week. Explain what you mean by fast food: meals bought from McDonalds, KFC, Burger King, Pizza Hut, etc. Tell them that fast food is not the same as high-sugar 'junk' foods like sweets or doughnuts, which have little nutritional value and will increase blood glucose levels very quickly when they are eaten. If you can discover which fast and junk foods your child is eating and when, all the better!

You may think that keeping food diaries is a lot of effort when you are already very busy but there is a good reason for it. Becoming aware of what needs to change and wanting to do things differently is the first important step on the journey to lasting change, known to health educators as the pre-contemplation phase. A reliance on sugar in the diet often involves denial in admitting what is being eaten, or even not being aware of you and your child's reliance on sugar. By doing a bit of food research, you are preparing the ground for how changes in lifestyle can be made and accepted. This is also preparation so your children will understand why, when you begin to make the changes to the family diet, this is happening.

TIP: _____

Give your children milk or water to drink at breakfast rather than fruit juice that is full of fructose with no fibre.

Think in terms of sufficiency, not deficiency and denial; you are adding nutritious, healthy foods to your child's diet before taking away the sugary snacks and drinks so they don't feel deprived. Sugary foods should not be removed from the diet until your children are enjoying their new diet and feeling better for it. Of course, you may be far keener to make a lifestyle change than your children are so be aware that you should go at their pace and not rush them. It may take eighteen months to get to where you want to be but eventually, with gradual small changes, you will achieve that goal: going at a slow pace allows the focus to be on the actual process rather than that you want your child and the whole family to be eating less sugar.

How to make a change to each meal

There are certain nutrients that you and your child need at each meal. Your body needs protein to build and repair tissues, make enzymes, hormones, and other body chemicals. Protein is an important building block of bones, muscles, cartilage, skin and blood, and is especially important in the diet of a growing child. Similarly, dietary fibre is needed for our digestive health and regular bowel movements. Fibre helps you feel fuller for longer, can improve cholesterol and blood glucose levels and can reduce the risk of developing diseases such as Type 2 diabetes, heart disease and bowel cancer.

Protein

Because children are growing, they need plenty of protein to form new body cells. This means that high-protein foods like meat, fish, cheese and eggs should be part of each meal. Dietary protein contains amino acids the body needs to produce enzymes and hormones, build muscle tissue, skin and bones and to transport nutrients. Children require more protein per kilogram of body weight than adults to support their faster growth rate. The amount of protein needed varies according to age, gender and activity level, as can be seen in the table opposite:

Age	Activity	Daily calories	Recommended daily protein	Protein per kg body weight
1–3 years	moderate	1,200	13g: 5–20% of daily calories	1.1g per kg
4–8 years	moderate	1,500	19g: 10-30% of daily calories	.95g per kg
9–13 years	moderate	1,800 for girls 2,000 for boys	34g: 10%–33% 34g: 10–30%	.95g per kg
14–18 years	moderate	2,000 for girls 2,600 for boys	46g: 10–30% 52g: 10–30%	.85g per kg

Making a game out of learning how much protein a child needs at each meal can be a good exercise. Use kitchen scales to see what 50g of grated cheese looks like or 80g of ham, but make sure it's just a game and that children don't then take it to the other extreme of weighing everything they eat. Your family will have certain things that they prefer to eat at each meal so I'm not going to suggest that you eat specific foods. When you go food shopping, involve your children and make a game out of checking the labels.

TIP: _____

Don't go shopping when you are tired and hungry, especially if your children go with you and they're feeling the same. You are more likely at these times to be attracted to sugary foods that can provide a glucose hit. Blood glucose levels will fall rapidly soon afterwards, so the effect is short-lived.

Eating protein-rich meals will help your child to stay full for longer, as well as being necessary for cell growth. If you are worried that your child isn't having enough protein in their diet you could add protein powder to meals that you cook yourself, but be wary of which ones you use. Daily consumption of soy-based protein powders can increase oestrogen levels in children: there have been cases reported of girls reaching puberty earlier and boys who have developed breast tissue. Whey protein powder is a good alternative.

Fibre

When fibre is part of a meal, blood glucose tends to remain stable rather than rising rapidly. Food manufacturers have realised that shoppers are looking for healthier products so they have increased the fibre content in some brands. As with alternative sweeteners, some types of added fibre are better than others and the best source is from eating vegetables and fruit. As we have seen though, the sugar found in fruit can also cause increased deposits of fat in the arteries if eaten in quantity because fructose stimulates the liver to produce fat, while the fibre content of fruit reduces this damage. This means that it is better to eat fruits such as pears and apples with the skin on than it is to eat a quantity of fruit with this fibre removed.

Fruit juice that has had the fibre removed or dried fruit that concentrates the sugars is high in fructose. Fruits that are high in fibre and contain the least fructose are cranberries, raspberries, gooseberries, blueberries and kiwi fruit. The fructose content of fruit and vegetables varies according to how old they are – think of how a new banana has a green skin and is hard and not very sweet, compared with a very ripe banana with brown marks on the skin that is sweet and soft.

TIP:

Don't forget that fruit juice is a concentrated form of fruit. A child might drink a small 250ml glass of mango juice while they would not eat two whole mangos. This illustrates the concentration of sugar found in fruit juice that is very easily transferred from the juice carton to your child's stomach. Remember, while fruit juice contains vitamin C, it has most of the healthy fibre removed.

General tips to reduce dietary sugar

Making the decision to reduce dietary sugar is not about avoiding sugar for evermore, it's about overcoming the constant desire for sugar so it becomes less important. Decide what you want to do first by order of importance and make that change gradually. Choose better alternatives and identify high-sugar foods containing glucose, dextrose, sucrose, white sugar, brown sugar, honey and syrup. Read food labels and be aware of less familiar sugars like microcrystalline cellulose – perhaps make a list of the less familiar ones and take it with you to the supermarket.

The carbohydrate content listed on food labels is a good indicator of the amount of hidden sugars in that food. If sugar is in the first three ingredients then that food or drink is not a good choice. Try to find snacks and desserts with a lower level of sugar as an alternative and remember, if 'natural' sugar appears on a food label it still contains sugar. I'm not suggesting you cut out all sugars, because that would be impossible. In the same way, I'm not saying always opt for low-fat, low-salt foods and avoid saturated fat and preservatives. Just be aware of the foods your family choose as knowledge is half the battle in making better choices.

Minimising withdrawal symptoms

Taking away the effect that sugar has on the brain also takes away the pleasurable feeling it delivers and has been delivering from birth, so it will be a shock to the system to correct this dependency – this should be done gradually. Going 'cold turkey' requires willpower to stop all forms of sugar in one go.

If you suddenly remove sugar from the diet, symptoms such as headaches, hunger, mild depression, emptiness and cravings are more likely. Cutting down on sugar but still having a significant amount means the craving is satisfied, but there is not enough sugar to cause a feeling of pleasure from eating it. Taking time to withdraw from sugar reduces the severity of withdrawal symptoms so that you may not experience any at all. The desire for sugar then disappears.

But this also means that eating something overly sweet in the future will reawaken the brain's connection and desire for sugar. Breaking the addiction means having a better control over the desire for sugar, not that it's OK to then eat it again.

The process of change allows for a backward step when we may slip up. It's human nature to do this and it's a very rare person indeed who makes a lifestyle change and then sticks to it for ever-more without wavering. If sugar has been reduced and then there's a slip up, for whatever reason, it will just mean that the process takes a little longer. A slip up should not be regarded as ruining weeks of healthier eating; it's not a big deal, as long as it doesn't happen too often to sabotage all the good work. If you withdraw from sugar over time, eventually the desire for it will diminish and then disappear.

TIP:

It is best not to go 'cold turkey' on sugar. Make gradual but progressive changes by choosing healthier alternatives.

Steve says, 'We had been eating a low-sugar diet as a family for about six months and we were all pretty well adjusted to it, feeling the benefits. My mother then came to stay and couldn't get on board with the idea, insisting we were depriving the kids of the treats they loved. This caused a lot of problems, especially when she took them out one day. When they arrived home the kids were hyper and edgy, not settling to anything and answering back, so we knew they'd had a lot of sugar. We said nothing but that night, my eight-year-old daughter told me she felt bad because they'd done something naughty. I guessed what was coming and told her it didn't matter, just this once. While I was annoyed that the kids had both eaten ice cream, sweets and cakes, followed by a huge Nando's dessert later on with all the sweet trimmings, there was nothing I could do. The kids both said they'd felt very sick and unwell but didn't want to upset Grandma. We sat down as a family the next day and talked about it. I think we have all learned a valuable lesson about sugar as the kids had to start almost from square one again as they had cravings for more.'

FACT: _____

Trying to cut a sugar habit by replacing it with alternative sweeteners is just as addictive because the brain is expecting something sweet.

There will come a day that even alternative sweeteners taste too sweet and you'll have no desire for sweet foods. Anecdotal evidence suggests that the withdrawal process takes longer and involves more sugar cravings for females compared with males, who seem to be able to achieve sugar withdrawal sooner and with fewer cravings along the way. If you are slowly reducing your child's sugar intake – and that of the rest of the family – make sure there is ongoing progress.

Obviously, gradual progress is more difficult to monitor over time than just cutting out everything in one go. If you convince yourself that it won't hurt to have an ice cream here or a bar of chocolate during the week, it's easy to slip back into addictive habits and not really be cutting down on sugar at all. Having the same amount of sugar in a cup of tea is another good example – gradually cut down over the weeks so that two spoons becomes one and then half a spoonful, until ultimately there is no sugar being added to tea because your taste buds have been trained to expect less. Keeping a food diary really helps to show progress and what's been achieved, as well as what was eaten and when, allowing you to keep motivated and on course with the lifestyle change.

In my book *How to Live Well with Diabetes,* I describe a way of eating for people with Type 1 diabetes called DAFNE, which stands for Dosage Adjustment For Normal Eating. It concerns being able to eat like a person who does not have diabetes so long as the right amount of insulin is given to manage blood glucose levels. In a similar way when you don't have diabetes, after adopting a low-sugar diet you can eat a wide range of healthy foods as long as they are low in sugar.

FACT: _____

If dietary sugars are reduced over time, the detoxification process becomes much simpler.

Caffeine and sugar

It is the case that human beings build up a tolerance to drugs like caffeine over time so more and more needs to be consumed to give us the same buzz. After drinking a cup of coffee or a Coke – even a diet version – the caffeine it contains takes up to an hour to have its peak effect, making us sharp and alert. Caffeine stays in our system for between three and seven hours, during which time it also passes into body fluids, which is why it is important to monitor your caffeine intake if you're pregnant or breastfeeding as it can reach the amniotic fluid in the womb and pass into breast milk. Caffeine also increases the heart rate because it causes a stress response in the body, as well as blocking the hormones that help us fall asleep.

When the diet consumed by either yourself or your child is high in caffeine, it has a profound effect. If we go back to the experiment showing that smaller bodies hold a greater concentration of sugar, the same goes for caffeine – it has a far worse effect on a child's body than on an adult who is larger. Caffeine disrupts the body's response to insulin, causing resistance so that more insulin is needed to reduce blood glucose to normal levels. This means that eating a high-sugar diet as well as drinking coffee and caffeinated drinks is a double whammy. This increased insulin response caused by caffeine or sugar is actually known as pre-diabetes and is what happens in children and adults who go on to develop Type 2 diabetes.

If your child is hooked on the caffeine and sugar in fizzy drinks then it's time to take action. Again, they won't be able to go 'cold turkey' straight away as sugar, caffeine and even artificial sweeteners are highly addictive substances. Gradually cut down on the amount you buy and make sure your child understands why they shouldn't buy them either. Replace with healthier alternatives like flavoured water and low-sugar fruit juices that are then diluted with some fizzy water before drinking as fruit juices contain a high amount of fruit sugar. Increase the fizzy water content of the drink until the drink contains very little juice and the majority is fizzy water.

FACT: _____

Pepsi has slightly more sugar, calories and caffeine than Coke. Coke has slightly more sodium (salt) than Pepsi. Next-generation vending machines are being introduced to dispense 200 variations of Coke tailored to consumer needs so it is possible to purchase a low-sugar, low-caffeine version, as well as changing the carbohydrate, potassium and sodium content.

FACT: _____

After the effects of sugar have left your child's system they won't miss it and they will find that eating something sweet doesn't make them feel as good.

Jay says, 'I started to cut the kid's sugar without them knowing, very gradually with less sugar on cereal and diluting fruit cordial with more and more water, then by swapping products for lower-sugar versions. After a couple of months, I told them what I'd been doing. They are eight and ten, so are old enough to see why I'd done it. They both said that they hadn't even noticed they'd been having less sugar and they got quite into the idea to see where we could cut out more. We've been looking at foods in the supermarket together and making smart choices for the whole family. I think this is something that many families could easily do.'

Making changes on a budget

You may be on a limited budget and need to be careful what you spend. The good thing about cutting down on sugar is that the money you don't spend on fizzy drinks and sweets can now be put towards other things like better wholegrain bread. I always used to think that heathy food was expensive food, and it can be when compared to the basic or value range most supermarkets offer. I studied my till receipts and marked what I considered to be foods that I didn't need to buy – things like crisps, biscuits and cake bought because members of my family wanted 'something nice' in the cupboard, or because visitors expected to be offered something along those lines. The total spend on junk food was an average of at least £10 per shop and I realised that I could get a lot of vegetables or bread for that money.

When you want to make a lifestyle change like reducing your family's sugar intake on a budget, do things slowly and plan what to buy before you go to the supermarket. You don't have to buy lean steak to have a healthier meal; chicken, eggs or canned tuna are good sources of protein. Make different choices such as buying porridge oats instead of sugary cereals. I know I have said that it helps to always include your child, but if you are at the very beginning of changing what you buy, it's better to go food shopping alone if possible so your child won't ask for sweets or their favourite sugary cereal. Take your time and search for supermarket own-brand alternatives that are cheaper than the branded varieties. If you compare the two you can often find that the own brand has less sugar or salt added. Take, for example, McVities digestive biscuits versus Asda own brand – and the own-brand are much cheaper too! You may find that taking the time to plan what you're going to buy for meals is one of the biggest changes you will make.

Opposition from others

Even though you're totally committed to reducing your family's sugar intake and you all understand why it's so important, you may face opposition from other people. Perhaps your own parents may feel that you are depriving their grandchildren by 'banning them from eating' sweet things. Your children may stay over with friends whose parents don't understand what you're doing.

I recall a school friend's mother giving me a sweet dessert because she 'felt sorry for me'. Now, I wasn't supposed to eat sweet things because of my Type 1 diabetes, but she didn't agree with denying a child a sweet treat. I refused the dessert, explaining why I couldn't have it. My friend's mother shook her head and said, 'Oh, one won't hurt!' My point is that many people outside of your home won't understand the concept of a low-sugar diet, so you need to develop some strategies before you are faced with this sort of situation. If your children are staying away from home, give them foods you're happy with and that they enjoy to take with them as an alternative. If you explain to other parents or relatives that there is a reason behind cutting the sugar – because it makes your child feel unwell with rapid swings in blood glucose – then hopefully they will understand and accommodate you by not offering your children really sweet 'treats'.

Colin says, 'A friend of the family could not see why we were trying to cut the amount of sugar our son was eating. The friend thought we were denying our son the treats he enjoyed and making life miserable for him but really, he had hyperactivity and we were trying to improve this. It was a difficult time and in the end, it was easier to drop the friend and do what was best for our son who is now so much better on a reduced sugar diet.'

Although it's been said that advertising only influences the brand of soft drink you buy rather than encouraging you to buy it in the first place, millions of pounds every year are spent by food manufacturers with adverts everywhere you look. For a family trying to turn away from the deeply embedded view that shows sugar as a source of comfort and love, this can be hard. It will take effort to explain to your parents that taking your child to the park is preferable to buying them sweets to show they care. Over time, you will become an expert in saying 'no' firmly but in a nice way. Your relatives and others will eventually notice the changes in your lifestyle and the benefits this brings, so your message will be reinforced.

Sugar is embedded in our lives in such a way that if we want comfort or are upset, we frequently turn to cake, ice cream, biscuits or chocolate because the brain then produces feel-good hormones. We traditionally offer sugary foods in celebration when the recipient is already happy that it's their birthday, wedding day or because they've achieved something amazing. Sugar can make us feel as though people care, giving sweet treats a high status when offering affection to others. Remember that the value is in the time you spend with people or doing things for them, and this counts far more than any cake or box of chocolates. Recall your childhood memories and the times spent with your parents or friends that you really enjoyed. The memories of seeing a great film at the cinema are not of the popcorn, they're of the occasion because you had a good time. Memories are made of events, not sweet treats.

KEY MESSAGES IN THIS CHAPTER

- It is possible to tackle a sugar habit in the same way as any addiction. A good way to start to reduce sugar intake is to cut down in stages rather than cutting it out of your child's life suddenly and completely.

- A manufacturer's serving may not be the same as what your child has been having – this may be closer to two or three servings in weight. To make your child more aware of what they're eating, play the game of measuring out grams of sugar to see what this really looks like.

- Replacing high-sugar foods with those rich in protein and good carbohydrates means that mood swings, temper tantrums, poor concentration and erratic blood glucose levels are eliminated.

- As part of the process of change, involve the whole family if possible and examine food labels. Be aware that this remains a fun, healthy activity for your child so it doesn't become an obsession with how many calories are being consumed.

- Think in terms of sufficiency rather than deficiency and denial so that you're adding nutritious, healthy foods to your child's diet before taking away the sugary snacks and drinks so they don't feel deprived.

- Reversing a sugar dependency should be achieved gradually. It requires willpower to stop all forms of sugar in one go, to go 'cold turkey'. If you stop sugar in the diet suddenly, symptoms such as headaches, hunger, mild depression, emptiness and cravings are more likely.

- When you want to make a lifestyle change like reducing your family's sugar intake on a budget, do things slowly and plan what to buy before you go to the supermarket.

- Sugar is embedded in our lives in such a way that if we want comfort or we're upset, we turn to something sweet because the brain then produces feel-good hormones. In the same way, sweet treats mark every life occasion and celebration. Memories are made of events, not sweet treats.

How Much Sugar Does That Contain?

There is so much nutritional information available now on food packaging and online that it can be difficult to know what to look for. The sugar content of foods, as with calories, fats and salt, is usually given per 100g of the product and also per portion. The difficulty lies in portion sizes varying from how much we eat ourselves or feed our children as we may consume two or three times more than the values provided. This chapter explains the sugar content of popular foods per 100g and, where appropriate, per bag or product so it's easier to see that some unexpected foods are very high in sugar. All values are accurate at the time of publication.

Bread

There are many types of bread available and in general the ones containing the least fibre tend to have a higher sugar content. For example, eating toast and sandwiches made from white bread can add up to three spoonfuls of sugar to the daily total. Products like bagels have a high sugar content as well – they are like doughnuts without the icing and filling – with 5.8g of sugar per plain white bagel, although a multigrain bagel contains only 3.4g of sugar. Multigrain, sourdough and rye bread has the lowest sugar content.

Unsurprisingly, what is spread on the bread can also make a big difference to sugar consumption. Many products designed to be spread on toast are aimed at children to encourage them to eat their breakfast if they're not having cereal. Needless to say, these products are generally high in sugar and while the adverts tell us that products like Nutella are great for giving kids energy in the mornings, this is because they're packed with sugar that will raise blood glucose levels rapidly, which will fall again by mid-morning. The amount of sugar consumed depends on how many slices of bread are eaten and how much of the product is used. Below is a list showing the average sugar content of products that can be spread on bread or toast, so always check the label.

Product	Sugar content
Honey	80 per cent sugar
Jam, marmalade and preserves	60 per cent sugar
Chocolate spreads	55 per cent sugar
Lemon curd	50 per cent sugar
Marshmallow spread	50 per cent sugar
Reduced sugar jams/preserves	45 per cent sugar
Reduced sugar peanut butter	30 per cent sugar

It's easy to see why sweet spreads like jam or marmalade would have a high sugar content, but some foods you might not expect, like peanut butter, can have sugar added to enhance their flavour. One hundred per cent whole nut butters are available in most supermarkets, but always check the label. The lowest sugar options are the savoury spreads such as Marmite, with less than half a gram of sugar per 20g serving. Soft cheese spreads also tend to be low in sugar, at around 3g of sugar per 20g, but again, always check the label to make sure.

FACT: _____

You will never be able to reduce the sugar content of the foods you buy to zero.

Breakfast cereals

Breakfast cereals were invented in the 1950s to make the first meal of the day quick and convenient. Children eat, on average, a 50g portion of breakfast cereal while an adult eats an average of 100g per bowl of cereal. By contrast, manufacturers tend to suggest a serving of around a quarter – 25g – of this amount. Most cereals, especially ones like Crunchy Nut Cornflakes, Frosties or Sugar Puffs are loaded with sugars, so any product above 3g of sugar per 100g should be treated with caution. Cereals with very little sugar – excluding the sugar you may add yourself – include Shredded Wheat, Weetabix original and plain porridge oats.

Product information gives the total sugar per 100g so it is easy to work out the percentage of sugar. For example, the list below shows that Froot Loops with marshmallows has 48.3g of sugar per 100g. This means that for every 100g of this cereal, 48.3 per cent is sugar. The following varieties of breakfast cereal contain the highest amount of sugar per 100g:

Kellogg's Froot Loops with marshmallows	48.3g
Kellogg's Smorz	43.3g
Kellogg's Apple Jacks	42.9g
Quaker Cap'n Crunch's Crunch Berries	42.3g
Kellogg's Froot Loops	41.4g
Kellogg's Ricicles	40.0g
Kellogg's Chocolate Cornflakes	39.0g
Kellogg's Frosties	37.0g
Kellogg's Honey Loops	36.0g
Dorset Berries & Cherries	36.6g
Nestlé Honey Cheerios	35.2g
Kellogg's Crunchy Nut Cornflakes	35.0g
Kellogg's Coco Pops	35.0g
Sugar Puffs	35.0g
Nestlé Oats and More (raisin)	31.8g

TIP: _____

Be aware of portion size: is the portion size suggested on the box the same as the portion size you or your child are consuming?

_____

It's the sugar that makes these products taste nice and it's the sugar that makes children – and adults – want them. You may think this leaves very little opportunity to carry on eating breakfast cereal as part of a reduced-sugar diet. That is certainly true for the list above and for supermarket own-brand varieties of these products. Always check the label and if sugar, glucose, fructose or honey is in the first three ingredients, avoid that product. There are breakfast cereals that are acceptable alternatives as long as table sugar, honey or fruit isn't added. The following is a list of breakfast cereals with a low sugar content per 100g unless otherwise stated:

Weetabix original (two biscuits)	1.7g
Mornflake oat bran	1.2g
Jordan's organic porridge oats	1.0g
Quaker Oat So Simple	1.0g
Ready Brek oat cereal	1.0g
Mornflake porridge oats	1.0g
Quaker porridge oats	1.0g
Scott's original porridge oats	1.0g
Nestlé Shredded Wheat original (two biscuits)	0.3g

Each of these breakfast cereals is low in sugar, fat, saturated fat and salt so they are healthy options.

Soft drinks

Soft drinks such as Coke contribute 10 per cent of the average child's daily sugar intake. As we have already seen, sugary soft drinks are especially damaging to a child's teeth, as well as providing a huge sugar hit in one go for a small person's body size. The best drink for a child's health is thirst-quenching water, which has the added bonus of being completely sugar-free! The next tooth-kind drink after water is milk, containing lactose (milk sugars). Lactose is less sweet than sucrose, but may be problematic for those with lactose intolerance. Milk is a rich source of nutrients in a child's diet, providing protein, calcium, potassium, iodine, phosphorus and vitamins B2 and B12.

Diet or low-sugar drinks such as squash with no added sugar or sugar-free lemonade have been sweetened artificially to make them palatable, but the artificial sweetener they contain will not help break a sugar addiction. These drinks are lower in calories than the sugary versions, so they don't contribute in the same way to weight gain. However, even if there is no sugar in a fizzy drink, the acid they contain to make them fizzy will still cause damage to teeth. In much the same way, fruit juice can cause tooth decay too. While a 150ml glass of no-added-sugar fruit juice provides vitamin C, it also contains fruit sugar which, although better than the sucrose or glucose that is added to drinks by manufacturers, is still sugar that will increase blood glucose levels.

A splash of full-sugar fruit squash or high-juice cordial diluted with water still provides around three teaspoons of sugar per 150ml glass, so it is not a healthy option as far as soft drinks go. The same goes for full-sugar fizzy drinks such as cherryade and ginger beer. These drinks, although better than Coke or non-brand cola which has added caffeine that children are more sensitive to than adults, are not healthy options because the combination of acid and sugar is damaging to teeth. A 330ml can of ginger beer contains 16g of sugar, while fizzy orange has 15g, with lemonade providing 14g of added sugar per can. A can of non-diet cola contains a massive 35g of sugar.

FACT:

The best drink for children and adults is water. A child's favourite soft drink is decided at an early age and children look to their parents to set a healthy example.

Energy drinks are not only expensive, but they do not provide more energy. In reality, a hit of glucose from one of these drinks causes a blood glucose spike, triggering insulin to be released by the pancreas in order to bring blood glucose levels back down to a normal level. Any sugary drink has the same effect, with a large insulin release potentially reducing blood glucose levels to lower than before the drink was consumed, causing tiredness and irritability. Zero-sugar energy drinks are sweetened with alternatives to sugar, so this contradicts the claim that these products provide a hit of energy for sports or as a pick me up. The energy from energy drinks comes from the glucose they contain.

The growing trend for fast-food outlets providing ice-cream milkshakes and 'freak-shakes' loaded with sugar from added biscuits, doughnuts, cake, cream, sweets and chocolates is – I'm sure I don't need to say – not a healthy choice. Additionally, these shakes decorated with all the trimmings can amount to 1,000 calories in one go – most children aged six to twelve should consume no more than 1,600–2,200 calories a day. Even as an occasional treat, freak-shakes are really unhealthy, causing a huge and sudden increase in blood glucose and blood fats.

The sugar content of some popular children's soft drinks is shown below:

Coke, 330ml	35g of added sugar
Copella apple juice, 300ml	31g fruit sugar (fructose)
Innocent orange juice with bits, 330ml	26g fruit sugar (fructose)
Ribena blackcurrant, diluted to 250m portion size	26g of added sugar
Innocent Smoothie, strawberries, blackberries and raspberries, 180ml	18g fructose from whole fruit and fruit juice
Fruit Shoot apple and pear, 200ml	15g fructose from fruit concentrates
Innocent juice tasty tropical, 180ml	14.4g sugar, contains fructose

Coconut water, 330ml	3.3g sugar, contains fructose
Fruit Shoot no added sugar apple & blackcurrant, 600ml	1.6g sugar and sweetened with acesulfame K and sucralose
Ribena no added sugar, diluted to 250ml portion size	1.3g sugar and sweetened with aspartame and acesulfame K
Robinson's squash no added sugar, diluted to 250ml portion size	0.3g sugar and sweetened with aspartame and saccharin

FACT:

Milkshake powders such as the strawberry and banana flavours produced by Nesquik contain 82 per cent sugar; the chocolate variety contains 77 per cent sugar. It's not just milkshake powders aimed at children that have a high sugar content. Meal replacement 'diet shakes' contain 50 per cent sugar too.

Fruit snacks

If you're trying to reduce your child's sugar intake, manufactured fruit snacks added to your child's lunch box or school bag are unfortunately not a healthy option as they contain an unacceptable quantity of sugars. Many 'healthy' fruit snacks aimed at children and labelled 'one of your five-a-day' contain more sugar than a bag of Haribo sweets. If the snack contains dried fruit then the fructose from the fruit will be concentrated, and the product will also contain sugar from other ingredients like honey, syrup and/or glucose that will have been added to the recipe to provide sweetness and bind the ingredients together.

TIP:

Fruit snacks and bars containing concentrated fructose from dried fruits score very high for sugars in a small snack. Instead of buying processed fruit snacks for your children that come with confusing and misleading information, give children fresh fruit and vegetables.

It is unlikely that you will measure out 100g of fruit snacks for yourself or your child to eat – amounting to four bags of pineapple pieces – so the following table shows the sugar content of popular fruit snacks, per bar as stated:

Whitworths Pineapple Pieces, per 25g bag	21.4g
Yu! Fruit Chews Strawberry, per 24g bag	20.9g
Fruit Bowl Yoghurt Raisins, one 30g bag	20.0g
Asda Yoghurt Flavoured Coated Strawberry Fruity Bits, one 25g bar	16.2g
Whitworths Sunny Raisins Coated Yoghurt Raisins, per 25g portion	15.8g
Asda Chosen by You Yoghurt Coated Raisins, 25g bag	15.2g
Fruit Bowl Blackcurrant Peelers, one 20g fruit peeler	12.0g
Fruit Bowl Strawberry Peelers, one 25g fruit peeler	12.0g
Fruit Bowl Strawberry Flakes, per 20g bag	12.0g
Frootz Blackcurrant 100% Fruit Drops, per 18g bag	11.0g
Frootz Strawberry 100% Fruit Drops, per 18g bag	10.6g
The Fruit Factory Fruit Strings: strawberry, apple & orange, per 20g bag	9.4g
Fruit Bowl Jungle Fruit Shapes, per 18g bag	9.0g
Kellogg's Strawberry Winders, one 17g winder	6.3g
Humzingers 100% Fruit Sticks, per 13g stick	5.0g
Bear Strawberry and Blackcurrant Pure Fruit Yo-Yos, per yo-yo	4.9g
The Fruit Factory Strawberry Fruit Wheels, one 15g wheel	2.7g

Each of the fruit snacks above is described by manufacturers as having no added sugar, which is true because they are naturally sweetened with fructose, but these snacks are not healthy alternatives to a chocolate bar.

Cereal bars

Cereal bars appear healthy because they are made with oats, fruit and nuts, but the reality is that most bars contain up to five teaspoons of sugar due to the fructose content of dried fruit. A two-finger Kit Kat bar, by comparison, contains two and a half teaspoons of sugar. Many cereal bars contain added sugars as well as fructose and lactose, so they are not necessarily a healthier alternative to a chocolate bar, even if they are marketed that way. Eating fruit and/or nuts in their natural form rather than in a processed cereal bar is the best option, especially walnuts, almonds and hazelnuts as these have proven health benefits. As cereal bars and biscuits are such an easy and popular lunch-box filler or portable snack food, here's a list of the sugar content in some of the most popular products:

Eat Natural Fruit and Nut Bars, per 50g bar	20.3g
Eat Natural brazil and sultana bar, per 50g bar	19.4g
Eat Natural dark chocolate, fruit and nut bar, per 45g bar	18.3g
Kellogg's Nutri Grain Biscuits, oat and chocolate chip bar, per 45g bar	17.0g
Alpen Trail Bar Big Berries, per 48g bar	14.0g
Belvita Breakfast Biscuits, one pack of 4 biscuits	13.0g
Kellogg's Nutrigrain Fruit Breakfast Bars (strawberry), per 37g bar	12.0g
Nature Valley Crunch (oats and honey), per 42g bar	11.9g
Jordan's Frusli (raisin and hazelnut), per 30g bar	9.6g
Kellogg's Coco Pops Snack bar, per 20g bar	8.4g
Kellogg's Special K Red Berry, per 23g bar	8.1g
Kellogg's Frosties Snack Bar, per 25g bar	8.0g
Tracker Crunchy Peanut Bar, per 26g bar	7.3g
Kellogg's Rice Krispies Bar, per 20g bar	7.2g
Jordan's Absolute Nut cereal bars, per 45g bar	7.2g
Quaker Oat So Simple morning bars (golden syrup), per 34g bar	6.1g
Harvest Chewee (milk chocolate chip), per 22g bar	5.9g

FACT:

Some cereal bars that are considered 'healthy' alternatives to conventional treats contain almost twice the amount of sugar as chocolate bars.

Cooking sauces and soups

It has always been assumed that eating foods with a high fat content makes us fat but research has now shown that it's the sugar in the diet and not the fat that is the problem. As I have mentioned previously, low-fat foods tend to have more sugar added than the full-fat versions of the same product as well as having more salt added to adjust for the increase in sugar. However, some manufacturers are realising that their customers want a healthier version of the products they enjoy. For example:

Heinz Cream of Tomato Soup 400g tin	Heinz No Added Sugar Cream of Tomato Soup 400g
Provides 19.4g sugar	Provides 10.6g sugar
8.6g fat	4.8g fat
2.2g salt	1.6g salt

Sharwoods Korma Cooking Sauce	Sharwoods 30% less fat Korma Cooking Sauce
¼ 420g jar provides 8g sugar	¼ 420g jar provides 6.3g sugar
8.4g fat	6.2g fat
0.7g salt	0.67g salt

Pasta sauce can contain as much sugar as a Mars Bar, with a 375g jar of Ragu smooth bolognese pasta basil sauce having 8g of sugar per 100g. To put this in perspective, that's 34 per cent of the daily recommended sugar intake for a child aged eleven years and older, 42 per cent of the recommended intake for a child aged seven to ten, and 53 per cent of the daily recommended intake for a child aged four to six.

REMINDER: The recommended maximum daily amount of sugars for anyone over the age of eleven is 90g. No more than 30g of this should be added sugar as opposed to naturally occurring sugars, such as fructose in fruit and lactose in milk. The NHS describes any product containing more than 22.5g of sugar per 100g as having a 'high' level, while anything below 5g is classed as 'low'.

FACT:
Ready meals are quick and easy but are often high in sugar to make them taste good. Always check the labels.

Tomato ketchup is a big favourite with children, but the reason it tastes so appealing is because ketchup contains 4.1g – one teaspoon – of sugar per tablespoon. Reduced-sugar versions have 50 per cent or less added sugar, but these can be more expensive. Check the labels and the cost and make the best choice available to you. If you have the time, you could make your own reduced-sugar tomato sauce or salsa – using tomatoes, onion, coriander and lime juice. There is a recipe for a healthier version of tomato sauce at the end of this book, and for those who prefer mayonnaise, there's a healthier recipe for that too.

Many popular brands of cooking sauces are high in sugar to enhance the flavour and give them bulk and 'mouth feel'. The sugar content per 100g of some of these products is shown below:

Sharwood's Hoisin Marinade Sauce	33.9g
Levi Roots Reggae Reggae Cooking Sauce	25.7g
Sharwood's Szechuan Kung Po Cooking Sauce	19.9g
Loyd Grossman Korma Sauce	8.9g

Ragu Red Sauce for Lasagne	7.6g
Ragu Smooth Bolognese Pasta Sauce	7.2g
Patak's Mild Korma Sauce	6.8g
Dolmio Bolognese Chunky Mushroom Pasta Sauce	6.6g
Dolmio Tomato Red Lasagne Sauce	6.4g
Loyd Grossman Tomato Roasted Garlic Pasta Sauce	6.3g
Dolmio Original Bolognese Sauce	5.8g
Homepride Pasta Bake Tomato and Pepperoni	5.1g
Loyd Grossman Tomato and Basil Sauce	4.8g

Soup is a quick and easy meal choice for lunch or dinner but with so many brands and flavours to choose from, it can be hard to work out which ones are healthy in terms of sugar content. Tomato soup tends to have a lot of added sugar to enhance flavour although, as we have already seen, Heinz now makes a no-added-sugar cream of tomato soup with 10.6g of sugar per 400g can compared to its full-sugar version at 19.4g per 400g can. The sugar content ranging from high to low of popular soups per 100g is shown below so that you can make an informed choice:

Crosse and Blackwell Tomato, 400g can	5.9g
Heinz Cream of Tomato with a Kick of Chilli, 100g can	4.8g
New Covent Garden Soup Co. Moroccan Tagine, 600g carton	4.0g
Asda Piri Piri Chicken Soup, 600g can	3.7g
Heinz Mulligatawny Soup, 400g can	3.3g
Heinz Farmers' Market Seven Vegetables Soup, 400g can	3.0g
Baxters Healthy Minestrone with Wholemeal Pasta, 415g can	2.6g
Heinz Cream of Mushroom, 290g can	2.1g
Asda Tomato and Red Pepper, 330g can	2.1g

Asda Spiced Pumpkin, 600g can	2.0g
Amy's Kitchen Hearty Rustic Italian Vegetable soup, 397g can	2.0g
Baxters French Onion, 400g can	1.8g
Weight Watchers From Heinz Carrot & Lentil Soup, 295g can	1.6g
Heinz Farmers' Market Broccoli and Stilton Soup, 400g can	1.6g
Asda Chicken and Sweetcorn Soup, 600g can	1.6g
Campbells Cream of Celery, 295g can	1.2g
New Covent Garden Soup Co. Leek and Potato, 600g carton	1.1g
Asda Oxtail Soup, 400g can	1.0g
Heinz Big Soup Smokin' Chicken and Bacon, 500g can	1.0g
Campbell's Cream of Chicken condensed soup, 300g can	0.8g
Baxters Pea and Ham, 400g can	0.7g
Heinz Big Soup Lamb and Veg, 400g can	0.5g
Baxters Scotch Broth, 400g can	0.4g
Heinz Chicken Noodle Soup, 400g can	0.1g

Pickles, sauces and dressings

It's not just sweet treats that provide a big hit of sugar. The majority of foods we eat have added sugars – pickles, chutneys and sauces being a prime example. While cooking sauces are eaten in a greater quantity than condiments such as tomato sauce per meal, it would be reasonable to think that a smaller quantity means less sugar. However, salad dressings can be anything from 0–20 per cent sugar, while the low-fat versions contain up to 5g more sugar per 100g than the full-fat version. While the amount of sugar consumed depends on the amount added to food, sauces like barbecue that don't taste overly sweet are up to 40 per cent sugar depending on the brand you buy; this is because the recipe also contains a quantity of salt to balance the sweetness. Below is a list showing the general percentage of sugar in the sauces we add to food, so look out for reduced sugar varieties.

Sauce	Percentage sugar
Sweet and sour	50
Sweet chilli	50
Plum	50
Barbecue	40
Worcestershire	35
Cranberry	35
Hoi sin	35
Ketchup	30
Apple	25
Fruity brown	25
Mint	20
Brown	20
Tartare	20
Chilli	20
Thousand Island/seafood	20
Low-sugar ketchup/brown	15
Horseradish	7
Mustard (not wholegrain)	5
Full-fat mayonnaise	4
Pesto	5
Taco	1.5
Soy	1
Tabasco	0

FACT:

While vinegar is generally free or very low in sugar content, Balsamic vinegar is a very concentrated, dark vinegar made from grape juice, seeds and stems. It contains 15g of sugar per 100g so adding it to salad dressings or cooking will increase the sugar content of the meal.

Manufacturers don't have to provide detailed nutritional content of the foods we buy in the UK unless that food claims to be a diet, low-fat or low-sugar version of a main product. It is unusual to find a food that doesn't have some nutritional information on the label these days, but the barest minimum is to list the calories, protein, fat and carbohydrate values only. The food label must list the ingredients in order of weight, so if some form of sugar appears as the first, second or third ingredient, you know the food is high in sugar. Look for the lowest-sugar versions of the product you can find and make the switch! Don't be fooled by products that are marketed and promoted as healthy or light versions. If a food is low-fat the manufacturers will have made up for the lack of flavour and volume with sugar to make the low-fat version appealing to the palate. If a snack food is marketed as healthy, check the label: *Go Ahead* products and anything involving dried fruit in the recipe, like muesli, contain 40 per cent sugar, sometimes more.

FACT:

Once you give up sugar, supermarket shopping is much quicker because you no longer visit the aisles containing biscuits and cakes, fizzy drinks and juices, or sweets and chocolate bars.

Yoghurts and yoghurt drinks

Flavoured yoghurts can be a minefield when you are trying to reduce sugar consumption. These products have increasingly been marketed as a health food for years but many, if not most, are more akin to a sweet dessert. In the UK, yoghurt appears in the top twenty favourite foods, with £1.7 billion spent each year on yoghurt and fromage frais. While natural and Greek-style yoghurts, which contain less sugar due to the way they are produced, are very healthy options in terms of fat and sugar content, flavoured yoghurts contain unhealthy levels of fat, sugar and food additives. While yoghurt is a product that naturally contains lactose, the majority of yoghurts and yoghurt drinks also contain added sugars from concentrated fruit syrup to make them an appealing product.

FACT: _____

Manufacturers group naturally occurring and added sugars together on product labels, shown as 'carbohydrates, of which sugars'. This makes it difficult to know whether a yoghurt is naturally sweetened with lactose and fructose only, or if sugars have been added by the manufacturer. The price of sugar and milk has fallen, making it cheaper for manufacturers to produce yoghurts with a high-sugar content.

Eating 'no added sugar' fruit yoghurts, although appearing like a healthy option, will increase blood glucose levels. Yoghurts are similar to fruity cereals and bars because they are sweetened with fruit concentrates or fruit juice extract, meaning they contain a lot of fructose. The manufacturer is right in saying that there's no added sugar in their product – meaning cane sugar – but this is misleading: for example, Total 0% Greek Yoghurt with honey has the equivalent of eighteen spoonfuls of sugar per 100g. All yoghurt products contain some lactose. Flavoured yoghurts should be swapped for plain, natural yoghurt if you want to reduce your child's sugar consumption.

Yoghurts and yoghurt drinks with a zero or low-sugar content per pot are listed overleaf:

Onken natural yoghurt	0 per cent sugar
Total Greek yoghurt	0 per cent
Actimel 0.1% raspberry	0 per cent – contains aspartame
Benecol strawberry yoghurt drink	0 per cent
Flora pro-active yoghurt drink	0 per cent
Weight Watchers berry fruits fromage frais	0.2 per cent – contains aspartame
Activia natural pouring yoghurt	0.2 per cent
Activia bio natural yoghurt	0.4 per cent
Weight Watchers confectionery yoghurts	0.4 per cent – contains aspartame
Weight Watchers citrus fruits yoghurts	0.5 per cent – contains aspartame
Benecol blueberry yoghurt drink	1.0 per cent
Benecol peach & apricot yoghurt drink	1.2 per cent

Once your family loses a taste for sugar you will find that sweet desserts don't have the same appeal. You will also feel satisfied with less food, so you just won't want to eat desserts or snacks. That may seem highly unlikely if you are just starting on the journey of a low-sugar lifestyle, but it really does happen. Food also becomes less of an issue and, to quote Benjamin Franklin, it is more important to 'Eat to live rather than live to eat': healthier foods encourage a longer life compared to eating a diet rich in unhealthy sweets and snacks. Eating these types of food feeds an addiction rather than a necessity.

Desserts found next to yoghurt in the supermarket chiller cabinet – especially the ones based on chocolate bars aimed specifically at children – are very high in sugar for their individual weight, as follows:

Cadbury Dairy Milk Daim dessert, 90g pot	26.2g sugar
Cadbury Dairy Milk buttons dessert, 90g pot	23.9g
Cadbury Crème Egg dessert, 90g pot	23.0g
Rolo Dessert, 70g pot	21.6g
Cadbury Flake dessert, 90g pot	20.6g
Müller Oreo Split Pot vanilla & cookie crumble, 120g pot	20.6g
Cadbury Dairy Milk dessert, 70g pot	17.2g
Aero milk chocolate mousse, 59g pot	14.0g
Milkybar white chocolate dessert, 70g pot	13.7g
Aero mint mousse, 58g pot	12.4g

A small pot of yoghurt may be 150g or 90g, so taking Rolo Dessert as an example, eating the whole pot would contain nearly eight teaspoons of sugar. If sugar appears first, second or third on the list of ingredients, the yoghurt is very high in sugar.

You will notice that some of the values given below are for a 450g pot, which would not be eaten as one portion. If a pot is eaten across two or three servings, this allows the sugar content to be calculated by dividing by one-half or one-third. Popular yoghurts with the highest sugar content per pot are shown here:

The Collective choccy orange yoghurt, 450g pot	75.0g
Yeo Valley 0% fat vanilla yoghurt, 450g pot	63.0g
Yeo Valley Greek style honey yoghurt, 450g pot	61.8g
Onken Greek Style apple and cinnamon yoghurt, 450g pot	25.2g
Activia fig yoghurt, 125g pot	20.0g
Müller Corner Fruit blueberry yoghurt, 150g pot	19.5g
Rachel's organic low-fat vanilla yoghurt, 150g pot	19.0g

Rachel's organic forbidden fruits peach yoghurt, 150g pot	18.5g
Müller Corner Crunch strawberry shortcake yoghurt, 135g pot	17.1g
Activia Fusions prune yoghurt, 125g pot	15.0g
Peppa Pig strawberry fromage frais, 45g pot	5.6g
Munch Bunch, 42g pot	5.2g
Wildlife Choobs, 40g tube	5.1g
Petit Filous strawberry & raspberry fromage frais, 47g pot	4.65g
Frubes, strawberry flavour, 47g tube	4.65g

TIP:

Don't forget that with a 450g family-sized pot of yoghurt, it's easy to eat more sugars in a portion size than in an individual 125g pot, unless you weigh out a 125g portion from the bigger pot.

Yoghurt drinks have become increasingly popular, with the added benefit that some contain probiotic live bacteria to encourage a healthy digestive system. These products are as healthy as they claim to be. Some yoghurt drinks include cholesterol-lowering plant sterols. While manufacturers promote yoghurt drinks as a healthy addition to your diet, some brands have a high sugar content per small bottle, as can be seen below.

Stonyfield low-fat organic strawberry smoothie, 170.48ml	24g
LALA Strawberry probiotic yoghurt, 198.90ml	16g
Chabani Drink mixed yoghurt, berry, 227.30ml	16g
Chabani Drink mixed yoghurt, strawberry & banana, 284.13ml	15g

Dannon Activia yoghurt drink, peach low-fat probiotic, 198.90ml	13g
GoGo Squeez Yoghurtz, banana, 85.25ml	12g
GoGo Squeez Yoghurtz, low-fat strawberry, 85.24ml	12g
Dannon DanActive probiotic yoghurt drink, strawberry, 85.24ml	11g
Dannon Light & Fit non-fat yoghurt drink, strawberry, 198.90ml	10g
Activia Yoghurt Drink, strawberry low-fat probiotic, 198.90ml	10g
Dannon Danimals Smoothie, low-fat strawberry explosion, 85.25ml	9.0g

Ice cream and ice lollies

You won't be surprised to hear that ice cream and fruit-flavoured ice lollies are also high-sugar products, so choose carefully if you are reducing sugar in your family meals. As with yoghurt and yoghurt drinks, ice cream is high in natural lactose and, depending on the recipe, additional cane or beet sugar, corn starch hydrolysate syrup, maltose syrup, fructose or high-fructose syrup, maltodextrin, dextrose, maple syrup or maple sugar, honey and brown sugar to enhance flavour. Don't be swayed by the claims of 'natural' sugars on boxes of ice lollies. This is just a marketing ploy. Fruit-flavoured ice lollies contain around 8g of sugar.

FACT: _____

Frozen yoghurt desserts aren't a healthier option over ice cream as both contain sugar from milk and fruit.

Making your own ice cream or ice lollies is the best option if you have the time. This way you can be sure there are no hidden extras like unlabelled sugars or preservatives added. If you are using an ice lolly mould, make lollies with sugar-free diluted cordial rather than fruit juice. Below is a list of some ice-cream brands available offering the most and the least sugar per 100g, which is one standard ice-cream scoop. As most adults and children will probably want to eat two scoops of ice cream for dessert, bear in mind that this means you need to double the values for sugar content in the right-hand column. Values are per 100g unless otherwise stated.

Cornetto Enigma vanilla and raspberry cone	28.3g
Ben and Jerry's Phish Food ice cream, 100g	27.3g
Nestlé vanilla and caramel cone	27.0g
Cornetto strawberry ice cream, 100g	25.3g
Ben and Jerry's Cherry Garcia ice cream, 100g	24.0g
Nestlé Rolo ice cream, per bar	19.7g
Kit Kat ice cream, per bar	19.6g
Cadbury Flake 99 cone	19.0g
Oreo Birthday Cake Ice cream, 100g	17.0g
Chapman's 97% fat-free frozen yoghurt, 100g	14.0g
Snickers ice cream, per bar	13.3g
Mars ice cream, per bar	12.4g

There is a recipe for low-sugar ice cream in the desserts section at the end of this book and you will find a recipe for reduced-sugar blueberry and avocado lollies in the snacks section too, for those who want to give it a go.

Eating out

Some fast-food restaurants, like McDonalds, provide detailed nutritional information online and in store about what goes into their food, so you can check the sugar content of your intended purchases, while Pizza Hut provides information online about balanced choices and meals under 550 calories. Provision of nutritional information is not generally available for Chinese, Indian, Thai or Mexican take-away or for fish and chip or pizza restaurants that are not part of a large chain, although it is worth asking or looking online. You don't need me to tell you that fast-food is not a healthy low-sugar choice to eat on a regular basis or even as a family treat. Thai or Malaysian food tends to contain more sugar than Chinese or Indian food, while pepperoni pizza is the lowest-sugar option compared with Hawaiian because of the pineapple. Frozen pizzas generally contain around 5 per cent sugar. Make home-made pizza or your own curries with curry powder and crème fraiche rather than curry paste or bought sauces, allowing you to reduce the sugar content.

Rob says, 'If possible, know what you want to order before you get to the restaurant so you can be sure of what you're eating. McDonald's is good because you can look up their nutrition information. It's easier to do this online at home rather than to try to work out what's low sugar when you have the kids with you at the counter and they're hungry. When we take the kids to an attraction, we take our own food as this is lower sugar and a lot cheaper. The kids will still want ice cream or candy floss if they see it for sale so we say they can have one treat and offer a choice of the smallest ice cream or a toy, not both. We tell them that the sweets are gone once they're eaten but they'll still have the toy. We never buy candy floss as it's made of pure sugar.'

KEY MESSAGES IN THIS CHAPTER

- Once you have gone through your shopping list and replaced high-sugar foods with lower-sugar alternatives, you will know which products to buy and your kitchen will only contain foods with the level of sugars you are happy with.

- Nestlé Shredded Wheat, Weetabix and porridge oats are low in sugar, fat, saturated fat and salt.

- Fruit snacks and bars containing concentrated fructose from dried fruits score very high for sugars in a small snack. Instead of buying processed fruit snacks for your children that come with confusing and misleading information, give children fresh fruit and vegetables instead.

- Some cereal bars that are considered as 'healthy' alternatives to conventional treats contain almost twice the amount of sugar as chocolate bars.

- Manufacturers don't have to provide detailed nutritional content of the foods we buy in the UK unless that food claims to be a diet, low-fat or low-sugar version of a main product. Check the ingredients list and if sugar or a form of sugar comes first, second or third, then that product is high in sugar.

Planning Low-Sugar Meals

Maintaining a reduced sugar lifestyle with a busy schedule can feel like a lot of effort. The key to managing your lifestyle change well is to plan ahead so you know what you will be eating each day of the week. This is also a great way to save money with low-sugar, nutritious and filling meals throughout your busy week. Keep in mind that your family will need foods rich in energy and protein to keep blood glucose levels stable.

Make your house as sugar-free as you can and make sure your children know why. Children are usually good at doing what they're told if they understand and respect the reason why. If they disobey they will feel bad about it, so buying chocolate or fizzy drinks on the way home from school or when they're out with friends won't become a regular thing to defy the rules, plus they'll remember what you told them while they're doing it. If your child tells you that friends have been eating something they particularly want to try, find it in the supermarket or online and read the label so you can decide whether the sugar content is acceptable or not.

Breakfast

Children probably won't refuse to eat the cereal you've given them if they are hungry. If your child refuses to eat their breakfast you could try the following: provide alternatives and let your child eat at their own pace; only give your child manageable amounts to eat, let your child decide when they are full and don't hover nearby, waiting for them to finish. In the case of a low-sugar cereal swapped for their favourite sugar-laden breakfast, they may choose to add sugar while they're adjusting to eating less. Don't worry if your child does add sugar to a low-sugar cereal like Weetabix, Shredded Wheat or porridge oats. The good news is that the amount of added sugar can be reduced over time if it comes from a bowl on the table rather than the set amount added to a sweetened cereal by manufacturers.

Blood glucose levels will have fallen during sleep so eating breakfast as soon as possible after getting up is essential after going for many hours without food. Your family may be very rushed in the mornings and leaving at different times so breakfast isn't always a priority. But eating something that will sustain you and your child until lunchtime and won't raise blood glucose levels rapidly is hugely important, especially when a child needs to be attentive during lesson time at school. Toast with jam and a cup of tea with sugar is not a healthy option. Don't ever miss breakfast and make it a must in your household: explain to your child when and why this change is going to happen so they know what to expect.

FACT: _____

Peanut butter is a very rich source of protein. Check the label on the brand you buy as some manufacturers put sugar into their peanut butter.

Anna says, 'Breakfast used to be a nightmare before we got into a low-sugar routine. Everyone wanted their sugary cereal as soon as possible and there were tantrums if they couldn't get what they wanted when they wanted. I cut the sugar down very gradually by swapping orange juice for milk and put a little sugar on cereal myself rather than letting the kids add it to their breakfast. They grumbled at first but soon got used to it. I then told them that their favourites weren't available and gave them a choice of Shredded Wheat or Weetabix. Because they had a choice rather than being told they had to eat one thing or nothing, they accepted it. I'm now working on lowering the amount of sugar in their packed lunches.'

Once everyone is on board with having breakfast because they know why it's important, the next issue is what to have. I've already mentioned avoiding sugary cereals as they don't provide a great start to the day. Alternatives need to be considered such as toast with Marmite or peanut butter for breakfast if there isn't time to make porridge or cook eggs, or if you know your children won't eat this. The last thing you want is a battle over food when you're hurrying to get ready in the morning. Decide at the weekend as a family that you are going to do things differently and discuss what kinds of foods everyone will eat so healthier decisions can be made. Ensure you have made these decisions together before implementing the change at the breakfast table. If you have a positive attitude towards a lifestyle change, your child will pick up on this and it will help adjustments to be made to your family routine each morning.

TIP:

Breakfast is non-negotiable but allow your children to have a choice in what they eat. The alternatives can be set by you to ensure the choice is healthier, so you could say, 'Marmite on granary toast or Weetabix?'

Hopefully, it won't be long before you see a difference once everyone is eating a better breakfast with more protein and less sugar. Having noticed changes in yourself and your child you may be tempted to introduce this sugar reduction into all your other meals straight away, but be patient. Get used to having a breakfast containing less sugar and more protein every day, and make sure you eat as soon as possible after waking up to stabilise blood glucose levels. Make this change first before you try to adapt other meals. You may find it hard to think of breakfast options if sugary cereal was the usual choice before your family started a reduced-sugar lifestyle. You could try some of the following blood glucose-friendly breakfast options, or you may already be eating something similar:

- Porridge with frozen blueberries or sliced banana added

- Cheese on wholegrain toast

- Scrambled eggs on wholegrain toast

- Wholegrain toast with cottage cheese and sliced tomatoes

- Wholegrain wraps with chicken or ham, cheese and tomato

- Peanut butter spread on a sliced apple

- Poached eggs on wholegrain toast

- Boiled egg with wholegrain toast soldiers to dip in

- Shredded wheat with blueberries or sliced banana added

- Banana and low-sugar/natural yoghurt smoothie made at home

Let your child decide what lower-sugar foods they would like to eat for breakfast and let them select these foods in the supermarket and put them in the trolley. If they are old enough, they may even want to have a go at making their own breakfast too.

Why do I need to eat breakfast – I don't want it!
Breakfast can be the last thing you want soon after you get up. Your brain can fool you into thinking you aren't hungry, even though your blood glucose is on the low side, and you can feel sick at the thought of food. This is because the body releases beta-endorphins to convince the brain that it doesn't need food as a protection measure. This hormonal response makes us feel that we don't need to eat. If breakfast is regularly skipped, this can be dangerous for children

because they are missing out on necessary proteins and vitamins needed for growth. For children and adults, eating in the morning is sometimes an effort, but feeling better afterwards is the reward as blood glucose levels stabilise.

Suzanne says, 'Breakfast was always a battle with my five-year-old daughter and she had an answer for everything. She wouldn't eat what she was offered and stomped around saying she wanted Sugar Puffs instead. If I explained why less sugar was important, she'd argue that her school friends were allowed to have whatever they wanted for breakfast. In the end, we decided to make changes to her diet where we could in evening meals and snacks rather than trying to change breakfast first, as she would refuse to eat anything if she didn't get her favourite. Eventually we calculated that her sugar intake had halved, so that was a major achievement. We cracked the breakfast problem on holiday abroad where my daughter could see there were no Sugar Puffs on offer so she had to compromise, even though she sulked about it. I think that because we'd not given up at the breakfast hurdle and we changed the amount of sugar in the rest of her diet, she was able to accept not getting the cereal she wanted.'

Your child may challenge what you say about the importance of eating breakfast without high levels of sugar with something like, 'Lisa's Mum says it's OK for her to have Coco Pops for breakfast!' or, 'Grandma has toast and marmalade, so why can't I?' Hopefully other members of your household will be keen to undertake and support the health benefits of cutting down on sugar. However, your child may see a different approach to breakfast when staying at a friend's home, or if there's a different family dynamic. Your answer will be that you are only responsible for your child's health, not Lisa's or Grandma's. It helps to tell other people about your sugar reduction, so explain to Grandma in advance and suggest breakfast options that you are happy with when your child spends time there.

TIP: _____
You need continuity to make any lifestyle change become a habit.

Lunch

As with breakfast, it is important for you and your child to eat a nutritious lunch. It's important to keep offering healthy lunch choices to your child as they learn to eat what is familiar to them; healthy food helps your child to concentrate and learn better at school. Set an example with your own lunches and encourage your child to choose and prepare their own lunch. They could also make a list of the foods they enjoy. It is important to offer fresh fruit, crunchy vegetables and a combination of protein, dairy and carbohydrates for lunches at home and in the school lunchbox.

TIP: _____
Sandwiches can be prepared in advance and frozen for school lunches.

Children need to eat something every three hours to keep blood glucose levels stable. It helps if they can eat at the same times each day. Discuss this with your child and find out what usually happens when they are at school during the lunch hour. If your child takes a packed lunch, making a change to reduce sugar will be much easier than if they eat school meals. If school lunches are on the menu, your child will need to know how to make healthier choices. If they think something might contain a lot of sugar, such as school desserts like gypsy tart or iced buns, both served up in local schools in my area, it is important to voice your concerns with a head teacher, or perhaps consider changing to packed lunches as a healthier option. Other issues also come into play, such as what your child's friends are eating for lunch and whether your child will follow their lead. The change in breakfast habits at home will train your child to know why sugar is an unhealthy option. Over time as your child's palate becomes more discerning they will want to eat healthier food, not things laced with sugar by the manufacturer to improve the flavour or texture.

FACT: _____

In the UK, around half of all primary school children have a packed lunch. Unlike school dinners, there are no official rules about what should be in a child's packed lunch to make them nutritious. A 2020 study found that ninety-eight out of a hundred packed lunches failed to meet nutritional standards. A child's packed lunch made with white bread, a cereal bar and a non-diet drink can contain the equivalent of fourteen teaspoons of sugar.

It may be the case that you also take a packed lunch to work with you. The same rules apply to this meal for adults and children. If eating out at lunchtime with colleagues, choose healthy, low-sugar options wherever possible. As most packed lunches for children and adults involve bread, be aware that white bread will raise blood glucose levels quickly once it's broken down, as will dense wholemeal bread. If possible, choose a bread that has seeds added to the recipe, like Hovis Seed Sensations, which is a great source of protein with seven seeds including brown linseed, sunflower seeds, pumpkin seeds, golden linseeds, millet and poppy seeds. This wholegrain bread is delicious and children really love it when it's made into toast or sandwiches. Molasses are added to the recipe so each 47g slice contains 1.8g of sugars; molasses count as a source of iron, so it is nutritious.

I know all these aspects of changing lifestyle require effort, but they really do pay off. I have previously mentioned the inclusion of whole grains in the diet to maintain steady blood glucose levels because they are healthier than refined foods. Avoid bread and pasta products made with white flour as they act in a similar way to sugar in the body to raise blood glucose rapidly. Look for alternatives such as wholegrain pitta breads that can be filled with protein and salad.

Dinner

A healthy evening meal is a must to provide the correct level of nutrition for adults and children. Dinner time should involve protein and as low a sugar content as can be achieved. Children can be involved in the process of shopping for food and choosing what they would like for dinner, but don't forget to offer two healthy choices so they think they've got their way. For example, you could say, 'Shall we have a cooked chicken from the supermarket with a baked potato and veggies or would you like wraps with home-made chilli?' If you change your approach it helps children accept the change. If a child is adamant about not eating what you're offering, suggest they try the food in question and if it isn't acceptable, promise to try something else in future.

TIP:

If you are too busy to cook in the evenings, you may rely on take-out or supermarket ready meals to feed the family, but it can be hard to know the sugar content of bought food. A roasted chicken from the supermarket is a good alternative and it goes a long way.

Depending on the age of your child you may want to involve them in cooking and preparing the food they eat so the whole process becomes something they enjoy. This also reinforces the lifestyle change as they are actively involved with reducing their sugar intake and eating better food. If a child prepares their own food – even part of it, like adding sliced banana to their cereal – they then feel that it's their food that they made, so they're more likely to eat it.

You may be faced with a child who 'dislikes' many foods, even if they haven't tried them! A nutritionist once told me that children will eat if they are hungry, but children can be very stubborn when they refuse to eat, sitting for hours at the table with arms crossed in defiance. This is a situation you don't need or want, and it might seem easier to give in. Your child may even ask, 'How much do I have to eat before I can leave the table?' Suggest a compromise rather than giving in completely or insisting that they have to finish everything on their plate. Agreeing that a child can leave the table but that they can't go to watch TV or play computer games while everyone else eats their meal works well, but the best way is to avoid these situations by giving your child meal choices. This way you can be more confident they will eat the meal, especially if they've been involved in the food shopping or preparation. Make dinner as relaxed and enjoyable as possible. If there are other adults in your household, ask them to support the reduced sugar message at mealtimes. Make sure everyone understands what you are doing and why it's important.

Pete says, 'My son is twelve and he refuses to eat certain foods because he doesn't like the feel of them in his mouth. At first, I thought he was just being picky, but I now know that this is a recognised condition called Avoidant Restrictive Food Intake Disorder. We have been working with a dietician and a child psychologist to get my son to try different foods such as carrots cut up to look like French fries. Over the past six months my son has gradually started to accept a few more foods. I'm hopeful that he will eventually be able to eat a well-balanced diet with the improvement he's making.'

Snacks

Make sure your child understands why it's healthier to eat snacks like peanut butter on a few wholegrain crackers instead of a couple of chocolate biscuits. Ask your child what they would like to take to school as a snack. A bag of crisps is a firm favourite but, again, check the labels for sugars and pick the best option – flavours like prawn cocktail and sweet chilli tend to be higher in sugar than other flavours. See if you can find vegetable crisps in the supermarket made from beetroot, parsnip and carrot; these look and taste good and are much healthier.

Dried fruit like raisins and apricots contain very concentrated fruit sugars, so eating these can be the same as a sugar hit from a doughnut. Fresh fruit still contains fructose, but just enough to boost your child's blood glucose until their lunch or main meal.

Don't give children under five years old whole nuts or peanuts as they may choke and are more at risk of an allergic reaction than older children. Crushed or ground nuts can be eaten instead.

> **Greg says,** 'As a child, I was labelled disruptive because I sometimes didn't pay attention and talked to other children in the classroom. I now recognise that this occasional behaviour was due to low blood glucose levels. Of course, when I was at school, the association between blood glucose levels and a child's attention span and performance in class simply weren't linked.'

Keeping a steady blood glucose level with regular meals and snacks containing necessary protein and carbohydrate rather than sugar is the key to achieving the right balance. Behaviour is adversely affected by high and low blood glucose in similar ways because too much or too little glucose irritates the brain, causing symptoms like irritability, short temper, tiredness and lethargy from low blood glucose levels; and hyperactivity, answering back, whinging, pouting, mood swings, shouting, and being stubborn or 'difficult' from high blood glucose levels.

FACT:
Having a glass of milk before bed can help stop your child's blood glucose level from falling too low over night.

When your child is at school you may feel powerless to do much about low blood glucose levels in the mid-morning after breakfast or in the afternoon once they've had their lunch. I certainly remember feeling very sleepy during the last lesson of the day – as did many other non-diabetic children in my class who were also flagging. It may be worth mentioning this to your child's teacher, although they will probably have already noticed that attention span can diminish before lunch and going home time. With the addition of a mid-morning and mid-afternoon snack of fruit – bananas are portable and excellent for this purpose – this will stop blood glucose falling and increase attention span.

TIP:
Your child needs a snack such as an apple or banana between meals – mid-morning and mid-afternoon – to keep blood glucose stable, especially if they are then walking home from school.

Soft drinks

Children are specifically targeted as customers by manufacturers of soft drinks like Coke or Pepsi. Not only is this product liquid glucose with ten teaspoons of sugar per can, it also contains high caffeine levels. Remember: both sugar and caffeine are highly addictive substances. Coca-Cola is never far away – whether at sports events, corner shops or vending machines – so it can easily be obtained by anyone addicted to it. Millions of pounds are paid every year by companies like Coca-Cola to sponsor sports or to support children's clubs and organisations so Coca-Cola can ensure an easy-access vending machine is always on hand. There are even vending machines dispensing Coke in schools and hospitals.

It is no wonder that it's so difficult to break the fizzy drinks habit when you consider the pervasiveness of brands like Coke and Pepsi in every part of our lives. It's not just children who enjoy the product, even if it's the diet version. It has been reported that Donald Trump drinks seven cans of Diet Coke every day. If you consider that a regular 330ml Coke has 35mg of caffeine per can and that Diet Coke has 45mg, Trump's intake amounts to 315mg each day – 400mg of caffeine per day has been deemed safe for a healthy adult. Adolescents aged twelve to eighteen should have no more than 100mg of caffeine daily – the equivalent of about one cup of coffee, one to two cups of tea, or two cans of Coke. For children under twelve, there's no designated safe limit.

FACT: _____

Roughly 73 per cent of children consume caffeine every day.

It may seem as though I'm demonising fizzy drinks when they are a big part of your child's life. The reason for this is that fizzy drinks are one of the largest sources of refined sugar in the average UK citizen's diet. Action on Sugar conducted a survey in 2014 to examine the amount of sugar being added to fizzy drinks by manufacturers.[1] They discovered the following shocking statistics:

- 79 per cent of sugary fizzy drinks contain six or more teaspoons of sugar per 330ml can – the World Health Organisation's recommended daily maximum for sugar.

- Nine out of ten sugary fizzy drinks would receive a red (high) traffic light for sugars.

- A typical can of cola contains as much sugar as three and half Krispy Kreme Donuts.

- Some elderflower sparkling drinks contain more sugars than Coke.

- 63 per cent of ginger beer drinks contain more sugars than Coke.

Tina says, 'I decided to go "cold turkey" on sugary drinks for the sake of my own and my daughter's health. It wasn't easy, but I poured what was in the cupboard down the sink. Once you've decided not to drink them any more you have to be firm – not, "We won't buy any more and just finish up this bottle." Be prepared for the challenge and have someone to discuss it with, although people don't tend to take fighting a fizzy drink addiction as seriously as quitting alcohol or cigarettes. My teenage daughter was my support and I was hers. Just having someone to say, "No" made all the difference. I did experience some headaches and my daughter felt tired because of the withdrawal, but nothing too serious. The sugar in these drinks can't be reduced gradually like in tea and coffee, so you have to cut them out. We didn't want to substitute diet drinks either because of the caffeine and additives, plus artificial sweetener doesn't allow you to stop wanting the sweetness of fizzy drinks. Cravings come from wanting these drinks because of the effect they have on our bodies, it's the desire for sugar in quantity. I'm pleased to say that we don't have sugary drinks any more and we are both now free of them.'

Holidays and celebrations

If you discuss what you are doing and why with your wider family, when there are get-togethers at Christmas, birthdays and other events everyone will be prepared and hopefully they will not offer your child sugary drinks or desserts. If you take your own food and drinks along to contribute to the occasion, it won't mean you are all sitting there wondering what to eat. I decided years ago that a good option for a family Christmas is to suggest we have a meal out at a restaurant rather than someone cooking. In this way, everyone can choose what suits them, avoiding any awkwardness. If it's your child's birthday and you know they love aeroplanes, arrange the day around a visit to an aircraft museum, or whatever interest they have rather than a party with sugary foods. If your child is enjoying the experience they won't be thinking about the lack of cake, sweets or Coke. Very young children won't know any better because they aren't expecting sweet treats on their birthday. I have even known a three-year old refuse to eat her birthday cake because it was too sweet. You can try making a low-sugar cake at home if you feel you must offer some sort of cake. There are some good low-sugar recipes online and

I've included a few at the end of this book. Remember that it's the time spent with people that matters, not the cake.

TIP: _____

If your child demands to try something new when you are in the supermarket, check the label together and decide whether the product is full of sugar, has a moderate amount of sugar, or no sugar or sugar alternatives. Your child may even start a new trend by taking a low-sugar drink to school and telling all their friends that it tastes great.

_____

If your child is attending a friend's party, the family hosting the occasion will be happy if you contribute some food for your child to take. You might want to ask before the event if there's anything your child can bring. If you are told, 'Just bring some crisps,' you can find a healthy version and send those along. If you're having a Halloween party, try hollowing out a pumpkin with your child so they can design the face, or make gift bags to give out filled with inexpensive things children will like such as stickers, fun-size bags of home-made popcorn, and so on. A friend of mine gives her children money rather than sweets so instead of having a pile of chocolate and sugary snacks, they can put the money towards the things they want.

If there's a big occasion coming up, make plans with your children before the event so they can make healthier choices. Cakes, sweets and fizzy drinks might be at the party but bringing tortilla chips with salsa dip, and flavoured sparkling water is a good compromise. Your child might not always make the healthier choice, but at least they're available.

Christmas

During Christmas, it's obviously not the best time of year to be starting a reduced sugar lifestyle, or at New Year when there may still be Christmas treats or sugary gifts from others in your household. If you do decide to cut down on sugar at Christmas but your children must have something sweet, let them have the treat after their main meal. The occasional sweet treat will still increase blood glucose rapidly but it's not as damaging to the body as eating lots of sugar each day. If your child eats their meal before the treat they are less likely to want a large quantity of chocolate or sweets. Keep treats in a cupboard rather than handing them out to eat later – sweet treats are the first thing on Christmas morning that your children will pounce on.

TIP:

Don't decide to start a sugar-reducing lifestyle change just before Christmas because it is stressful enough without worrying about what you can eat.

Gary says, 'It's so easy at Christmas to eat too much sugar because there are sweets and chocolates on the sideboard and before you know it, the kids have eaten half a tin of Quality Street. Last year, I decided to make a change and not buy any additional treats because I knew the kids would receive a selection box or two as presents. I put them in a cupboard with a lock on it and just allowed the kids to have one bar of chocolate each on Christmas afternoon in front of the TV after they'd had their Christmas dinner. It worked really well because the treats weren't just there to be picked at without thinking. Leaving it all out on display sends the message that they can dig in when they want!'

Easter

At Easter, focus on doing craft activities with your children rather than giving them lots of chocolate. Decorate the shells of some hard-boiled eggs together on Maundy Thursday that you and your child can then have for breakfast on Good Friday, or hide the decorated eggs around the house so they can have an egg hunt. Again, if you are just starting to cut down on sugar, a small chocolate egg can be a treat after the main meal is eaten, but avoid Cadbury Creme Eggs as they are filled with very high-sugar fondant as well as the chocolate casing. As with all childhood and happy family memories, the good times you have together are the important thing, not the chocolate. Make chocolate less of a focus.

There are many other religious holidays and festivals not mentioned here. The same principles apply and your sugar-reducing skills are transferable to any occasion where food is part of the celebration. Plan well and discuss what you are going to eat with your family before the event. Be prepared that other people may ask questions or try to force sweet things on you or your child because they either don't understand or they don't agree that reducing sugar is important. If you are in the first few weeks or months of reducing sugar, choose foods that are lower in sugar than those you would normally be eating, or reduce the amount of sugar added to what you cook.

TIP:

Remember, reducing sugar in the diet is a gradual process and behaviour change only happens over time.

Parties

When your child goes to a party they will be faced with an array of sugary choices. Finding the right balance between eating well and not sticking out like a sore thumb is something that will come in time but as long as your child knows that party snacks are not everyday foods because they are only to be enjoyed now and again, that is a good start to reducing overall sugar consumption. If your child has been eating less sugar for a while they will really notice how sweet many party foods are anyway, so they will make their own decisions. Older children especially will realise that they are not enjoying that cupcake covered in thick icing, so they won't want a second one. Allow your child to make their own food choices where possible – which you will have to do anyway because you won't be with them at school or parties or sleepovers – within the guidelines you have given them for staying away from sugar. There are some recipes for low-sugar party foods at the end of this book.

Kim says, 'I've always provided savoury snacks to send with my kids to parties so I think people are just used to that now. I don't think anyone expects loads of cakes and sweets as families are far more health-conscious now, so they're looking for healthier alternatives. This goes for the kids too; my children hate really sweet things and ask me to make low-sugar birthday cakes and snacks because they just don't enjoy all that sugar. Hopefully, people's tastes are changing as they realise that they need to make healthy choices.'

KEY MESSAGES IN THIS CHAPTER

- Make your house as sugar-free as you can and make sure your children know why.

- Eating breakfast within an hour of getting up is essential after going for many hours without food while sleeping as blood glucose levels will have fallen overnight.

- You need continuity to make any lifestyle change become a habit. Explain what you are doing and why to relatives and friends so they can support you.

- Don't decide to start a reduced-sugar lifestyle change just before Christmas because it is stressful enough without worrying about what you can eat.

- Remember, reducing sugar in the diet is a gradual process and behaviour change only happens over time.

Recipes

Hopefully by now you will have adjusted to a lower-sugar lifestyle. As we have seen, it's impossible to completely remove sugar from your family diet without growing everything yourself and making each meal to ensure not a grain of added sugar or any of its alternatives gains entry to your kitchen.

I have included here some low-sugar recipe ideas for breakfast, lunch, dinner, dessert, snacks and treats that I find taste better than the full-sugar versions and some that don't include sugar at all. Some of the recipes do have a small amount of sugar added, but these dishes are considerably lower in sugar than any bought, manufactured brand.

Eating is all about choice: you may not wish to make your own ice cream or reduced-sugar fruit cake – even if the sugar content per slice is only 4.3g – once you have lost your taste for sweet things and kicked your sugar addiction. I have included cake and biscuit recipes so they are there if you want them. Your family may have only started to reduce sugar a few months before the festivities so you feel you want something in the house that is a lower-sugar alternative to a bought Christmas cake, or you just want something healthier to offer visitors.

Whatever your situation, enjoy experimenting with reduced-sugar recipes and even try to cut sugar in your meals further so you and your family are eating as little sugar as possible. If your children are old enough, involve them in cooking the foods they will be eating. Just a word of warning: obviously don't use any of the following recipes if they contain ingredients that you or your family are allergic or intolerant to.

If you are home-baking, instead of relying on sweetness in the recipe, try experimenting with vanilla or almond extract, or ginger, cinnamon or nutmeg to enhance and add new flavours. Finally, enjoy your food and your low-sugar lifestyle and remember that it is not about denying certain foods or dieting, it's about finding acceptable and healthier alternatives!

Recipes sourced from: https://www.diabetes.org.uk/guide-to-diabetes/recipes

Potato patties

MAKES 12
Preparation time: 10 minutes
Cooking time: 25 minutes
Each pattie provides 9.6g carbohydrate; 67 calories;
less than 0.5g sugars; 1.8g fat; 0.2g salt.

Ingredients:
450g potatoes, peeled and chopped
3 egg whites, whisked to soft peaks
Freshly grated nutmeg, to taste
A little sunflower oil, for frying
Salt and freshly ground black pepper

Method:
1. Boil the potatoes for 10–12 minutes, or until soft. Drain and mash well, or press through a potato ricer. Leave to cool completely, then stir in the beaten egg yolks and nutmeg and season well with salt and pepper.

2. Gently fold the whisked egg whites into the potato mixture. Heat a little oil in a non-stick frying pan, form the mixture into twelve patties and cook in batches until golden brown on both sides.

3. Set aside each batch on a piece of kitchen paper to absorb any excess oil and keep them warm until you're ready to serve.

Tasty toasties

SERVES 4

Preparation time: 10 minutes

Cooking time: 10 minutes

Each toastie provides 35.3g carbohydrate; 294 calories; 3.3g sugars; 11g fat; 1.6g salt; 1 portion of vegetables.

Ingredients:

1 wholemeal baguette, cut into sixteen 1.5cm-thick slices

8 cherry tomatoes, halved

1 red pepper, cored, seeded and thinly sliced

4 mushrooms, sliced

1 slice of lean ham, cut into strips

70g cooked spinach, water squeezed out

2 spring onions, finely sliced

2 eggs, scrambled

75g reduced-fat mature Cheddar cheese, finely grated

Method:

1. Heat your grill to medium and toast the baguette slices until golden on both sides. Allow to cool. (You could use the cooling time to prepare your toppings, if you haven't already.)

2. Use the remaining ingredients other than the cheese to top the slices of baguette – combine them according to your taste and preferences, making a few options.

3. Sprinkle each topped slice with a little grated Cheddar, then place them back under the grill until the cheese is golden and bubbling. Serve immediately.

Mini berry pancakes

MAKES 10 PANCAKES
Preparation time: 10 minutes
Cooking time: 15–20 minutes
Each mini-pancake (74g) provides 16.3g carbohydrate; 100 calories;
2.8g sugars; 1.8g fat; 0.2g salt; ½ portion of fruit.

Ingredients:
200g wholemeal flour
1 tsp baking powder
1 medium egg, beaten
250ml skimmed milk
1 tsp vanilla extract
200g blueberries
2 tsp sunflower oil
1 tsp sugar substitute
Lemon juice

Method:
1. Mix the flour and baking powder in a bowl.

2. In a separate bowl, beat together the egg, milk and vanilla extract.

3. Make a well in the middle of the flour, then gradually stir in the egg and milk mixture until you get a smooth batter.

4. Ideally, leave to stand for a few minutes before cooking.

5. Lightly crush half the blueberries with a fork and mix these into the batter along with the remaining whole blueberries.

6. Add a little oil to a non-stick frying-pan, then add the batter to the pan making sure the blueberries are evenly distributed.

7. Cook the pancakes on a medium heat for 2–3 minutes then turn them and cook for a further 2 minutes. The pancakes will be ready to turn when you see bubbles appearing on the surface. Sprinkle with a little sugar substitute before serving with a dash of lemon juice.

Avocado, banana and pumpkin seed toast

SERVES 4

Preparation time: 5 minutes

Cooking time: 3 minutes

One-quarter (110g) of the avocado mixture on one slice of wholegrain toast provides 316 calories; 25g carbohydrate; 9g protein; 18g fat; 7.4g sugars; 0.4g salt; 1 portion of fruit and vegetables.

Ingredients:

75g pumpkin seeds

4 slices wholegrain bread

1 large avocado

1 large banana

Method:

1. Remove the skin and stone from the avocado and peel the banana, placing both in a bowl.

2. Toast the bread and divide the four slices diagonally, or slice into toast soldiers.

3. Mash the avocado and banana together in a bowl using the back of a fork, then blend in the pumpkin seeds, keeping some back to sprinkle over the mixture for decoration.

4. Spread the mixture on the toast and sprinkle with the remaining pumpkin seeds.

Cream cheese and tomato bagels

SERVES 2
Preparation time: 10 minutes
Cooking time: 10 minutes
One toasted wholemeal bagel provides 357 calories; 63g carbohydrate;
7.7g fibre; 17.7g protein; 3.3g fat; 9g sugars; 1.6g salt.

Ingredients:
4 medium tomatoes, halved
1 tsp sunflower oil
2 wholemeal bagels
60g fat-free Quark soft cheese
Freshly ground black pepper to taste

Method:
1. Under a heated grill, place the halved tomatoes on a baking tray with the cut side downwards. Grill for 3 minutes before turning to grill the other side for 3 minutes until slightly browned on both sides.

2. Slice the bagels in half and toast them, then spread with cream cheese. Place three tomato halves on one bagel half. Top with another half bagel and do the same for the second bagel.

3. Top both completed bagels with a little more cream cheese and remaining tomato halves and sprinkle with black pepper to taste.

TIP:
You could use cottage cheese instead of Quark and grilled mushrooms instead of tomatoes.

Walnut and apricot granola

SERVES 10
Preparation time: 10 minutes
Cooking time: 25 minutes
Each 52g serving excluding any added milk provides 185 calories;
25g carbohydrate; 3.3g fibre; 6.1g protein; 6g fat; 4g sugars; 0.01g salt.

Ingredients:
1 tsp rapeseed oil
300g jumbo oats
35g pumpkin seeds
35g walnut pieces
1 egg white, beaten
3 tsp alternative sweetener
75g raisins
75g apricots, chopped

Method:

1. Preheat oven to 150°C/Gas mark 2 and use the rapeseed oil to grease a large baking tray.

2. In a bowl, mix the oats, seeds and walnuts. Set aside.

3. Lightly beat the egg white with alternative sweetener until frothy. Add the egg to the oats, seeds and nuts in the bowl and ensure that everything is well coated.

4. Spread the mixture evenly onto the baking tray and bake for 15 minutes.

5. Add the raisins and apricots and mix them well on the baking tray. Bake for a further 10 minutes.

6. Leave the granola on the baking tray to cool.

TIP

The granola can be kept in an air-tight container for up to two weeks.

Cheesy breakfast burritos

SERVES 8
Preparation time: 10 minutes
Cooking time: 10 minutes
Two burritos provide 391 calories; 37.7g carbohydrate; 7.4g fibre; 19.3g protein;
16.4g fat; 3.7g sugars; 1.4g salt; 1 portion of vegetables.

Ingredients:
8 wholemeal tortillas
2 large tomatoes, chopped
1 red pepper, sliced
4 spring onions, chopped
100g frozen spinach, defrosted and drained
1 avocado, peeled and sliced
80g Cheddar cheese, grated

Method:
1. Prepare the fillings.

2. Place tortillas in a stack in a frying pan over a low heat with no oil. Turn them regularly so each side becomes warm but not toasted. Heat tortillas in rotation until all have been warmed through but not crisped.

3. Remove the tortillas from the heat and place separately on a clean work surface. Cover the bottom half of each tortilla with some of each of the fillings, except the grated cheese.

4. Sprinkle the grated cheese over the ingredients in each tortilla and roll it, tucking the sides in.

5. Place the rolled tortillas into a frying pan with no oil, seam side down, and cook for a further two minutes, turning them a couple of times to make sure they are evenly cooked.

TIP:
You can wrap these burritos in greaseproof paper so your child can eat them in the car. You could also fill the tortillas with scrambled eggs and mushrooms for a low-sugar breakfast or lunch, although this changes the nutritional values given above.

Coronation chicken salad

SERVES 4

Preparation time: 30 minutes

Each serving provides 450 calories; 10g carbohydrate; 40g protein; 3g fibre; 5g sugars; 30g fat; 0.6g salt.

Ingredients:

375g cooked chicken, cubed

3 hard-boiled eggs, chopped

3 heaped tbsp low-fat mayonnaise

1 tbsp curry powder, or to taste

½ tsp garlic powder

298g tin apricots in natural juice, drained and chopped

4 small spring onions, chopped

60g fresh coriander, chopped

60g pecans or almonds, chopped

Salt and black pepper to taste

Method:

1. Mix all of the ingredients together in a large bowl and serve immediately, or refrigerate and use within two days. Serve with green salad or as a sandwich, wrap or wholegrain pitta filling (salad or bread suggestions not included in the calorie total for this dish).

Cheddar and mushroom omelette

SERVES 1
Preparation time: 5 minutes
Cooking time: 10 minutes
The omelette provides 251 calories; 3g carbohydrate; 2.5g sugars; 16.5g fat; 0.7g salt; 2 portions of vegetables.

Ingredients:
2 eggs
Pinch of white pepper
1 tsp sunflower oil
150g mushrooms, sliced
1 spring onion, chopped
10g reduced-fat Cheddar cheese

Method:

1. Break the eggs into a bowl, add the pepper and beat with a fork. Set aside.

2. Heat the oil in a frying pan and cook the mushrooms and spring onion for 5 minutes on a medium heat, stirring regularly until soft.

3. Stir the eggs into the mushrooms and spring onion, then cook gently for 3 minutes. Use a spatula to ease the omelette from the sides of the frying pan.

4. When the omelette is cooked, sprinkle the cheese on top and slide it out onto a plate, folding it in half so that the cheese is in the middle.

Tuna and onion salad

SERVES 2
Preparation time: 5 minutes
Half (453g) of this salad provides 330 calories; 22.6g carbohydrate; 12.3g fibre;
32g protein; 9.8g fat; 7.4g sugars; 0.2g salt; 4 portions of vegetables.

Ingredients:
1 red onion, finely chopped
180g cherry tomatoes, halved
8cm cucumber, cubed
150g salad leaves
400g tin chickpeas in water, drained (240g)
200g tin tuna chunks in water, drained (150g)
20ml olive oil
Grated zest of half a lemon
Black pepper to taste

Method:

1. Grate lemon zest into a large bowl and add black pepper and olive oil.

2. Add red onion, tomatoes and cucumber and mix well.

3. Mix in chickpeas and tuna chunks so all ingredients are coated with the salad dressing.

4. Add the salad leaves to the bowl and divide the salad between two lunch boxes or bowls.

TIP:

You could also use prawns in this salad but make sure that if it's going in a lunch box, this does not get hot in the sun. Packing this salad lunch with a frozen low-sugar drink in the morning will keep the tuna or prawns nicely chilled and fresh until lunchtime.

Leek and goat's cheese quiche

SERVES 4
Preparation time: 15 minutes
Cooking time: 35–40 minutes
Each 150g serving provides 150 calories; 12.5g carbohydrate; 2.4g fibre;
9g protein; 6.5g fat; 2.3g sugars; 0.3g salt; 1 portion of vegetables.

Ingredients:
1 tbsp rapeseed oil
320g trimmed leeks, chopped
5 squirts olive oil spray
2 sheets filo pastry cut into 4 squares (80g)
2 eggs, beaten
2 tbsp 0 per cent fat Greek yoghurt
30g goat's cheese
1 tbsp chopped chives
Generous grind black pepper

Method:
1. Preheat oven to 180°C/Gas mark 4.

2. Over a low to medium heat, pour rapeseed oil into a saucepan and add leeks.

3. Spray a flan dish with oil then spray each pastry square, arranging them in the flan dish to create a star shape.

4. In a bowl, beat eggs, yoghurt and black pepper. Stir in softened leeks and place the mixture into the flan dish. Sprinkle goat's cheese over the top and bake for 15 minutes, or until centre of the quiche is just set.

5. Garnish with chives and a little black pepper before serving.

TIP:
You could use broccoli instead of leeks. This quiche can be frozen after cooking and defrosted when required, reheating thoroughly before eating.

Chicken and salad tortilla wraps

SERVES 2
Preparation time: 20 minutes
Cooking time: 10 minutes
A serving of 1½ tortilla wraps (356g) provides 454 calories; 52.7g carbohydrate; 15g fibre; 32.4g protein; 9.3g fat; 7.8g sugars; 0.9g salt; 3 portions of vegetables.

Ingredients:
1 tsp olive oil
1 small onion, chopped
1 red pepper, sliced
1 skinless chicken breast, sliced
400g tin red kidney beans (240g rinsed, drained)
1 tbsp low-fat crème fraiche
3 small wholemeal tortillas
1 small carrot, peeled and grated
60g salad leaves
Black pepper to taste

Method:

1. Heat the olive oil in a non-stick pan and add chopped onion and sliced pepper. Fry for 2–3 minutes until soft. Add the chicken slices and cook for a further 3–4 minutes until brown and cooked through.

2. Mash together kidney beans and crème fraiche in a bowl. Warm the tortillas for a couple of minutes in a dry pan with no oil, changing the position of bottom tortilla to top until all three are warmed through.

3. Divide the bean mixture between the tortillas and add the cooked chicken. Sprinkle each tortilla with grated carrot, salad and seasoning to taste. Roll tortillas and serve.

TIP:

You could use mushrooms instead of chicken for a veggie wrap. These tortillas can be frozen and used at a later date.

Creamy bacon and leek pasta

SERVES 2
Preparation time: 10 minutes
Cooking time: 12 minutes
Each serving provides 472 calories; 71.6g carbohydrate; 20.7g protein;
6.9g fibre; 9.8g sugars; 8.2g fat; 0.9g salt; 1 portion of vegetables.

Ingredients:
175g dried pasta shapes
2 rashers of lean back bacon, chopped
1 leek (about 150g), finely chopped
1 tsp chopped rosemary
1 small carton of natural yoghurt
1 tbsp sun-dried tomato paste
Freshly ground black pepper, to taste
A little grated Parmesan, to top
Salad vegetables, such as cherry tomatoes and rocket leaves to serve

Method:

1. Cook the pasta according to packet instructions, then drain and set aside.

2. Meanwhile, place the bacon into a frying pan and dry-fry for 2 minutes. Add the leeks and rosemary and fry for a further 3–4 minutes, until the leeks are cooked.

3. Mix together the yoghurt and sun-dried tomato paste and stir into the cooked pasta, adding the bacon, leeks, rosemary and black pepper to taste. Sprinkle a little Parmesan cheese on the top and serve with plenty of salad vegetables.

Mini bacon and rosemary muffins

MAKES 48 MINI MUFFINS OR 18 LARGER MUFFINS.
Preparation time: 20 minutes
Cooking time: 15–20 minutes
Two muffins (24g) provides 60 calories; 8.3g carbohydrate; 0.4g fibre;
1.9g protein; 2.2g fat; 0.4g sugars; 0.2g salt.

Ingredients:
250g plain flour
250g fine polenta
1 tbsp baking powder
1 tsp paprika
350ml milk
750g reduced fat spread such as Flora Light, melted
2 eggs, beaten
2 rashers back bacon, grilled and chopped into small cubes
2 tsp fresh rosemary, chopped
2 tbsp fresh Parmesan cheese, grated

Method:

1. Preheat oven to 200°C/Gas mark 6. Lightly grease your muffin tin. Mini muffins need to be made in batches unless you have several tins.

2. In a large bowl, sieve flour, polenta, baking powder and paprika and mix well.

3. In a separate bowl, blend milk, reduced fat spread and eggs before folding into the dry ingredients. Add the bacon and rosemary and mix well.

4. Spoon appropriate amount of mixture into tins depending on the size and quantity you are making. Sprinkle each muffin with a little grated Parmesan cheese.

5. Bake for 8–10 minutes until golden brown. Cool before serving or serve slightly warm if preferred.

TIP:

These are great for lunch boxes. You could make a veggie version using sun-dried tomatoes instead of bacon. These muffins can be cooked and frozen. Defrost for 2 hours.

Easy tomato sauce

An easy tomato sauce for pasta and home-made pizzas
that can be stored in the freezer.

SERVES 4
Preparation time: 5 minutes
Cooking time: 5 minutes
Each 55g serving provides 20 calories; 3.8g carbohydrate; 0.6g fibre;
0.8g protein; 3.6g sugars; 0.01g salt.

Ingredients:
½ medium onion, peeled and finely chopped
1 clove of garlic, peeled and finely chopped
200g chopped tomatoes, tinned or fresh
2 tsp tomato puree
2 tbsp cider vinegar
1 level tsp dark muscovado sugar

Method:

1. Place the ingredients in a small saucepan.

2. Simmer for 5 minutes.

3. Purée and set aside to cool.

Garlic and red pepper mayonnaise

MAKES 300G

Preparation time: 15 minutes

Cooking time: 30 minutes

One tablespoon of mayonnaise contains 28 calories; 1.6g carbohydrate; 1.9g fat; 1.3g sugars; 0.1g salt

Ingredients:

100g fat-free, natural fromage frais

55g onions or shallots, sliced

55g reduced-fat mayonnaise

1 red pepper, cored and chopped

1 large clove garlic, peeled

1 tsp olive oil

Small handful fresh basil

Method:

1. Preheat oven to 220°C/Gas mark 7. Put onions, red pepper and garlic into a small roasting tin and drizzle over the oil. Making sure everything is coated in oil, cook for 20–30 minutes, or until contents of the roasting tin are soft and golden brown. Add the fresh basil in the final 10 minutes of cooking time.

2. Leave mixture to cool, then blend with the fromage frais until smooth. Add the mayonnaise and refrigerate in a covered container or jar.

TIP:

Keep this mayonnaise in the fridge and eat within three days of making.

Garlic roast potatoes

SERVES 4
Preparation time: 5 minutes
Cooking time: 50 minutes
One-quarter of this dish contains 310 calories; 5g protein; 55g carbohydrate;
3g fibre; 3g sugar; 10g fat; 0.89g salt.

Ingredients:
4 large (225g) Albert Bartlett or Desiree potatoes, unpeeled
2 tbsp olive oil
½ tsp granulated garlic powder
2 garlic cloves, crushed
Salt and black pepper to taste

Method:
1. Preheat oven to 200°C/Gas mark 6.

2. Scrub potatoes and cut into 2-inch cubes.

3. Mix garlic powder, salt and pepper with olive oil and toss the potato cubes in the mixture.

4. Place potato chunks onto a lightly oiled baking tray and cook for 45 minutes, stirring occasionally.

5. Add crushed garlic to potatoes and toss to coat the chunks evenly. Return to the oven and cook for a further 5 minutes until garlic is cooked through and potatoes are soft and golden brown.

Beef goulash

SERVES 2

Preparation time: 15 minutes

Cooking time: 3 hours 5 minutes

One serving provides 370 calories; 36.6g carbohydrate; 12.7g sugars; 8.7g fat; 1.7g salt; 2½ portions of vegetables.

Ingredients:

250g lean braising steak, diced

250g new potatoes

2 tsp seasoned plain flour (use black pepper and a salt substitute to season)

1 tsp sunflower oil

1 onion, chopped

½ red pepper, chopped

1 garlic clove, crushed

1 tsp paprika

200g tomatoes, chopped

1 tsp tomato purée

150ml beef stock

Method:

1. Preheat oven to 180°C/Gas mark 4.

2. Toss the steak in the seasoned flour. Heat the oil in a flameproof casserole dish, add the steak and fry for 2–3 minutes until brown all over.

3. Add the remaining ingredients and bring to the boil, then put the lid on the casserole dish and place in the oven for 3 hours, or until the meat is tender.

4. Serve with plenty of vegetables.

Sweet potato fish pie

SERVES 6
Preparation time: 10 minutes
Cooking time: 45–55 minutes
Each serving provides 339 calories; 36.9g carbohydrate; 12.8g sugars;
8.4g fat; 0.9g salt; 2 portions of vegetables.

Ingredients:
1kg sweet potatoes, peeled and chopped
1 tsp sunflower oil
2 leeks, halved lengthways, then sliced
1 heaped tsp plain flour
1 fish stock cube
400ml skimmed milk
Good pinch of white pepper
25g parsley, plus extra to garnish
1 heaped tsp paprika
300g skinless, boneless pollack, cubed
300g skinless, boneless salmon, cubed
Pinch of black pepper, to serve

Method:

1. Preheat the oven to 180°C/Gas mark 4. Cook the sweet potatoes in a pan of boiling water for 15–20 minutes until soft, then drain.

2. Meanwhile, heat the oil in a saucepan and fry the leeks, stirring regularly until soft, about 7 minutes.

3. Sprinkle the flour over the leeks and crumble the stock cube over. Mix well for a minute to coat the leeks.

4. Slowly stir in 100ml of the milk, until the leeks are coated in a thick paste, then gradually add in the remaining milk, stirring constantly until the mixture comes to the boil. Stir in the white pepper and parsley and remove the pan from heat.

5. Mash the sweet potatoes until smooth and stir in the paprika.

6. Add the leek sauce to an ovenproof dish and arrange the fish so that it's evenly distributed over the top. Top with the sweet potato and bake for 25–35 minutes, until the sauce starts to bubble through the sweet potato. Sprinkle with parsley and black pepper.

Enchanting enchiladas

SERVES 4
Preparation time: 10 minutes
Cooking time: 30 minutes
One-quarter of this dish provides 470 calories; 58g carbohydrate; 14g fibre;
25g protein; 12g fat; 18g sugars; 2g salt; 4 portions of vegetables.

Ingredients:
2 tsp olive oil
2 small onions, chopped
2 cloves garlic, crushed
250g mushrooms, sliced
1 pepper, chopped
1 carrot, grated
2 tsp chilli powder, to taste
1 heaped tsp oregano
1 heaped tsp cumin
2 tbsp tomato purée
400g tin chopped tomatoes
400g tin mixed beans, drained and rinsed
400g tin green lentils
4 x 65g large wholemeal tortillas
200g low-fat plain yoghurt
75g low-fat cheddar

Method:
1. Preheat oven to 180°C/Gas mark 4. Heat oil in a saucepan and fry onion until soft. Add the garlic, pepper, mushrooms, chilli powder, oregano and cumin. Mix ingredients together and cook until soft.

2. Add tomatoes, tomato purée and carrot; mix well. Bring to the boil then reduce heat. Cover with saucepan lid and simmer for 10 minutes, stirring occasionally.

3. Add mixed beans and green lentils. Mix together and bring to the boil. Stir and remove from heat.

4. Spread 4 tbsp of the mixture over the base of a large ovenproof dish. Place 4 tortillas on a work surface and divide the mixture equally between each. Fold in the ends and roll each tortilla, placing them in a row in the dish.

5. Mix the plain yoghurt and grated cheese and spread over the enchiladas. Bake in the oven for 15 minutes until golden brown. Serve with either salad vegetables or rice (not included in calorie/carbohydrate value given).

Cheesy spinach cannelloni

SERVES 6
Preparation time: 5 minutes
Cooking time: 25 minutes
Each serving provides 160 calories; 20g carbohydrate; 4.8g fat;
5.5g sugars; 0.3g salt; 1 portion of vegetables.

Ingredients:
120g dried (not pre-cooked) cannelloni pasta
1 tsp sunflower oil
1 large onion, finely chopped
1 leek, finely chopped
3 garlic cloves, crushed
250g frozen leaf spinach
150g ricotta cheese
½ tsp nutmeg
400g tin chopped tomatoes
1 tbsp oregano
1 tbsp tomato purée
A generous grind of black pepper
25g mozzarella cheese, thinly sliced

Method:

1. Preheat the oven to 180°C/Gas mark 4.

2. Add the oil to a saucepan and cook the onion and leek for 5–8 minutes. Mix in the garlic and cook together for another couple of minutes, then remove from the heat.

3. Add the spinach, ricotta cheese and nutmeg to the pan and mix well.

4. Put the tomatoes in a bowl and add the oregano, tomato purée and black pepper. Mix together to make the sauce.

5. Stuff the spinach and ricotta mixture into the cannelloni. Put half the tomato sauce in an ovenproof dish. Place the stuffed cannelloni on top and add the remaining sauce. Top with mozzarella and bake for 15 minutes until golden and bubbling.

Mini baked potatoes filled with salmon and horseradish

Preparation time: 15 minutes
Cooking time: 40 minutes
Each 63g mini potato provides 80 calories; 8.3g carbohydrate; 1g fibre;
3.5g protein; 0.8g fat; 1.2g sugars; 0.1g salt.

Ingredients:
12 small potatoes (500g)
4 tbsp fat-free fromage frais
2 tbsp horseradish sauce
1 tbsp fresh chives, chopped
50g tinned salmon
Freshly ground black pepper, to taste

Method:
1. Preheat oven to 200°C/Gas mark 6. Prick the skin of each potato a few times and place on a baking tray. Bake for 35–40 minutes.

2. Blend the fromage frais and horseradish in a bowl.

3. Cut halfway into each potato so that it opens up.

4. Spoon a little of the fromage frais and horseradish into each potato. Top each potato with a little salmon, and black pepper to taste, and garnish with chives before serving.

TIP:
You could use chunks of tuna or strips of ham, beef or chicken as a source of protein, or add cooked mushrooms in place of the fish or meat.

Chicken curry

SERVES 4
Preparation time: 20 minutes
Cooking time: 35 minutes
One-quarter of the curry provides 330 calories; 32g carbohydrate; 5.5g fibre;
36g protein; 5.3g fat; 9.3g sugars; 0.3g salt; 3 portions of vegetables.

Ingredients:
1 tsp ground cumin seeds
1 tsp coriander seeds
1 tbsp rapeseed oil
4 medium onions, thinly sliced
4 cloves garlic, thinly sliced
2 green chillies, opened
½ oz fresh ginger, finely grated
400g chicken breast, cut into small chunks
½ tsp chilli powder
1 tsp garam masala
1 tsp turmeric powder
400g tin chopped tomatoes
150g tin lentils
Juice of a lemon

Method:
1. Put the cumin and coriander seeds in a dry saucepan and heat for 1–2
minutes. Add the rapeseed oil and sliced onions, cooking for 5 minutes
and stirring regularly until the onions are browned.

2. Add the green chillies, garlic, ginger and chicken chunks and cook for
a further 2–3 minutes, stirring regularly.

3. Add the chilli powder, garam masala, turmeric powder, lemon juice,
chopped tomatoes and 500ml of water to the pan.

4. Stirring regularly, bring to the boil, then reduce heat and simmer for
15 minutes.

5. Add lentils and simmer for a further 15 minutes, stirring regularly until cooked. Serve with rice or quinoa but remember that the nutritional information is for the curry only and not any additions.

TIP:

Instead of using individual spices to flavour your curry, you could use curry powder or curry paste but check that the paste does not have added sugars. This curry can be stored in the freezer once cooled. Defrost in the fridge rather than in the microwave and ensure curry is cooked thoroughly as you are reheating chicken.

Tender sage pork and vegetables

SERVES 4
Preparation time: 10 minutes
Cooking time: 1¼ – 1½ hours
One-quarter of this dish provides 185 calories; 6.1g carbohydrate; 28.6g
protein; 4.3g fat; 5.7g sugars; 1.1g salt; 2 portions of vegetables.

Ingredients:
300g Savoy cabbage cut into wedges
8 baby leeks, trimmed
1 bulb fennel cut into wedges
½ tsp sage
Pinch of white pepper
1 vegetable stock cube dissolved in 400ml boiling water
1 tsp rapeseed oil
4 lean pork steaks (300g)
3 tsp Dijon mustard

Method:

1. Preheat oven to 170°C/Gas mark 3. Arrange the vegetables in an ovenproof dish and sprinkle with sage and pepper. Pour the vegetable stock over.

2. Pour the rapeseed oil into a hot pan and add pork steaks; cook for 1½ minutes on each side to brown.

3. Place the pork steaks over the vegetables in the ovenproof dish and spread with a little of the mustard.

4. Cover the dish tightly with kitchen foil and bake for 1¼–1½ hours. After 1 hour, check that the dish still has stock – if not, add a small amount of hot water.

TIP:

You can also use skinless chicken or turkey breasts, or lamb steaks for this recipe although the calorie values will be slightly altered.

Apple and carrot bake

SERVES 4
Preparation time: 10 minutes
Cooking time: 40 minutes
One-quarter provides 270 calories; 6g protein; 35g carbohydrate;
9g fibre; 12g sugars; 14g fat; 0.43g salt.

Ingredients:
Roughly 0.5kg carrots, peeled and cut into 1-inch cubes
Roughly 0.5kg apples (not cookers), unpeeled, cored and cut into cubes
118ml unsweetened apple juice
1 tbsp olive oil
½ tsp cinnamon, or to taste
2oz toasted almonds

Method:

1. Preheat oven to 190°C/Gas mark 5. Lightly oil a 33 x 23 x 5cm baking tray.

2. Mix all of the ingredients except the toasted almonds and place in prepared pan.

3. Cook for 40 minutes, or until carrots and apple are soft and golden brown.

4. Sprinkle over the almonds and serve hot.

Berry and vanilla trifle

SERVES 10
Preparation time: 25 minutes, plus 2 hours cooling
Cooking time: 15 minutes
Each serving provides 120 calories; 9g carbohydrate; 4g sugars;
6.8g fat; 0.2g salt; 1 portion of fruit.

Ingredients:
For the sponge
40g wholemeal flour
½ tsp baking powder
5 tsp granulated sugar substitute
2 tbsp light olive oil, plus a little extra for greasing
1 small egg, beaten
1 tsp of vanilla extract
50ml water

For the custard
250ml skimmed milk
20g cornflour
1 tsp vanilla extract
5 tsp granulated sweetener
2 tsp semi-skimmed milk

For the jelly
1 x 23g sachet of sugar-free strawberry jelly crystals
300g frozen mixed berries

For the topping
200g low-fat Greek yoghurt
200g half-fat crème fraiche
10g toasted flaked almonds
Grated zest of 1 lemon

Method:

1. To make the sponge: in a bowl, mix together the flour, baking powder and sweetener. Add the 2 tablespoons of oil, the egg and the vanilla extract and mix thoroughly until smooth.

2. Add 50ml of water and beat. Lightly oil a 570ml microwave-proof bowl and pour the mixture in.

3. Microwave on full power – 800 watts – for 2 minutes and 20 seconds, then allow to cool.

4. To make the custard, put the milk in a saucepan and bring to the boil.

5. Meanwhile, put the cornflour, vanilla extract, sweetener and 2 teaspoons of semi-skimmed milk in a cup and mix well until smooth.

6. Once the milk is about to boil, add the cornflour mixture, stirring continuously with a wooden spoon and bring to boiling point, stirring until thickened. Remove from the heat and leave to cool.

7. To assemble, break the sponge into pieces and scatter on the bottom of a glass bowl.

8. Make the jelly according to the packet instructions, but use 10 per cent less water than stated. Set aside and allow to cool for 10 minutes.

9. Scatter the frozen berries on top of the sponge, then pour the jelly over the fruit and sponge and place in the fridge for 30 minutes to set.

10. Spread the custard over the jelly and return the trifle to the fridge for 30 minutes. Cover with cling film and refrigerate until you're ready to serve (overnight if you wish).

11. To finish the trifle, mix the yoghurt and crème fraiche together and use this to top the custard, then scatter with almonds and lemon zest.

Christmas pudding

SERVES 8
Preparation time: 15 minutes
Cooking time: 1 hour 15 minutes
One-eighth of the pudding (66g) provides 130 calories; 22.4g carbohydrate;
3.2g fibre; 2.7g protein; 2.8g fat; 10g sugars; 0.1g salt; 1 portion fruit.

Ingredients:
25g currants
25g raisins
25g sultanas
10g mixed peel
1 tbsp mixed spice
1 tbsp ground cinnamon
½ tsp ground cloves
½ tsp ground ginger
½ tsp olive oil
20g glacé cherries, chopped and washed, leaving 5 whole cherries for decoration
10g whole almonds
1 small banana
1 small unpeeled apple, grated
1 small carrot, grated
50g fine oatmeal
30g wholemeal flour
½ tsp baking powder
Zest of 1 lemon, grated
Zest of 1 orange, grated
10g sunflower seeds
10g pumpkin seeds

Method:

1. Preheat oven to 180°C/Gas mark 4. Boil 50ml water in a kettle.

2. Place all the dried fruit in a large bowl, mixing thoroughly. Pour over the 50ml of boiled water and cover the bowl with a tea towel for 15 minutes.

3. Brush the olive oil around a 1-pint pudding basin and arrange the 5 whole cherries and some whole almonds on the bottom of the basin for decoration.

4. Using a separate bowl, mash the banana and mix with the grated apple, grated carrot, oatmeal, wholemeal flour, baking powder, fruit zest and seeds.

5. Add the spices, fruits soaked in boiling water and the soaking water to the mixture, stirring everything thoroughly before adding the mixture to the pudding basin.

6. Cover the top of the basin tightly with pleated greaseproof paper and kitchen foil.

7. Place the pudding basin in a deep oven tray containing 5cm water and bake for 1 hour.

8. Remove the oven tray and lift out the pudding basin. Place pudding basin back in the oven for a further 10 minutes then remove from the oven but keep the cover on. Allow to cool for 10 minutes before serving.

TIP:

You could use 75g of mixed dried fruit rather than buying currants, raisins and sultanas separately. If you don't have ginger, cloves and cinnamon, add an additional 2 tsp of mixed spice to the recipe. This pudding mixture can be frozen before the Christmas holidays so it is ready to cook nearer the time, or it can be frozen once cooked, then heated in a microwave or steamed once defrosted.

Paradise rice pudding

SERVES 4
Preparation time: 3 minutes
Cooking time: 30 minutes
Each serving provides 179 calories; 32g carbohydrate; 6g sugars;
4g fat; 0.3g salt.

Ingredients:
100g basmati rice
400ml tin reduced-fat coconut milk
300ml soya milk
25g caster sugar or 2 dessertspoons of granulated artificial sweetener
Few drops of vanilla extract
1 tbsp toasted coconut

Method:

1. Place all the ingredients except the toasted coconut into a small saucepan. Place over a low heat and simmer very gently for 20–30 minutes until the rice is tender.

2. Transfer to a serving dish, top with toasted coconut and serve.

Blueberry cheesecake

SERVES 12
Preparation time: 18 minutes / Cooking time: 12 minutes
Freezing time: 4 hours
Each 120g serving provides 150 calories; 16g carbohydrate; 2g fibre;
9.4g protein; 5.2g fat; 5.8g sugars; 0.4g salt.

Ingredients:
For the cheesecake base
150g rolled oats
1 tbsp wholemeal flour
1 tbsp granulated sweetener
4 tbsp sunflower oil

For the topping
450g blueberries
2 tbsp lemon juice
2 tbsp granulated alternative sweetener
500g 0 per cent fat Greek yoghurt
250g 3 per cent fat cream cheese, such as Philadelphia low-fat soft cheese

Method:

1. Preheat the oven to 180°C/Gas mark 4. Grease and line a 20cm tin with baking parchment.

2. In a large bowl, mix together all the ingredients for the base. Press the mixture firmly into the base of the baking tin.

3. Bake for 10–12 minutes until golden brown on top. Leave to cool.

4. For the topping, blend around one-quarter of the blueberries with the lemon juice and one tbsp granulated sweetener.

5. Pass topping through a sieve into a large mixing bowl. Add the Greek yoghurt, cream cheese and remaining sweetener, mixing well.

6. Spread evenly onto the cooled base and top with remaining blueberries. Cover and freeze the cheesecake for 4 hours.

7. Remove from the freezer about 45 minutes before serving to soften it.

8. Remove from tin and cut into slices with a warm, damp knife.

Summer fruit Eton mess

SERVES 6
Preparation time: 20 minutes
Cooking time: 1 hour 45 minutes
Each 120g serving provides 85 calories; 12g carbohydrate; 2g fibre;
8g protein; 0.3g fat; 5.6g sugars; 0.2g salt.

Ingredients:
4 tbsp water
3½ tbsp granulated sweetener
1 tsp lemon juice
6 egg whites
1 tsp cream of tartar
4 tsp cornflour
400g fresh fruit
200g 0 per cent fat Greek yoghurt

Method:
1. Add water, lemon juice and granulated sweetener to a small saucepan over a low heat until the liquid becomes like a syrup.

2. Place egg whites and cream of tartar in a bowl and whisk slowly until the mixture forms soft peaks.

3. Gently add the syrup from the saucepan to the egg white. Add cornflour and fold in until egg whites become stiff.

4. Line a baking tray with parchment and arrange or pipe the meringue to form a 25cm-wide bowl shape.

5. Bake at 100°C/Gas mark ¼ for 1 hour 20 minutes, or until firm. Open the oven door and leave baking tray inside until meringue is cool.

6. Place the cooled meringue in a bowl and cut into bite-size pieces. Roughly mix the meringue pieces, fruit and yoghurt and serve.

TIP:
If the meringue starts to brown before it's ready, open the oven door to reduce the temperature.

Apricot and orange delight

SERVES 6
Preparation time: 10 minutes
Cooking time: 20 minutes
One-sixth (113g serving) provides 144 calories; 17g carbohydrate;
1.7g fibre; 3g protein; 6.6g fat; 10g sugars; 0.1g salt.

Ingredients:
2 x 300g tin apricots in natural juice
1 large orange using zest and juice
50g rolled oats
25g flaked almonds
15g butter, melted
1 tbsp sesame seeds
1 tbsp runny honey

Method:

1. Preheat oven to 200°C/Gas mark 6.

2. Using an ovenproof dish, make a single layer of apricots. Drizzle orange juice and zest over the top and cook for 10 minutes.

3. Meanwhile, mix together oats, melted butter, almonds, sesame seeds and honey for topping in a bowl.

4. Spoon topping over the apricots and return to oven for 10 minutes, or until golden brown.

TIP:

You could also use peaches in this dessert. This can be served with crème fraiche, but remember that this isn't included in the nutritional information.

Strawberry and banana ice cream*

SERVES 8
Preparation time: 2 hours
Cooking time: 10 minutes
*For this recipe, you will need a pre-chilled ice-cream maker.
One-eighth of this ice cream contains 285 calories; 9g carbohydrate; 1g fibre;
4.5g protein; 26g fat; 8g sugars; 1 portion fruit.

Ingredients:
300ml double cream
300ml whole milk
1 vanilla pod cut lengthways with seeds removed or 2 tsp vanilla bean paste
6 large free-range egg yolks
500g fresh strawberries, halved with stalks removed
100g ripe banana, peeled weight

Method:
1. Add cream and milk to a large saucepan and stir in the vanilla pod with seeds or your vanilla paste. Bring to the boil then immediately remove pan from the heat.

2. In a large bowl, whisk egg yolks until pale, then whisk in cream and milk. Return the mixture to the saucepan and place over a very low heat.

3. Heat for around 5 minutes, stirring constantly until the mixture looks like custard and it's thick enough to coat the back of a spoon. Be careful not to overheat the mixture, otherwise the eggs will scramble.

4. Remove the custard from the heat and take the vanilla pod out; pour into a clean bowl. Cover the bowl with cling film to prevent the custard forming a skin and leave to cool.

5. Blend strawberries and banana to a purée in a food processor or with a handheld blender. Mix the fruit purée with the cooled custard and pour into a pre-chilled ice-cream maker. Churn for up to 30 minutes until thick before transferring to a freezer-proof container. Freeze until the mixture is solid.

6. Remove from the freezer and leave to stand for 10 minutes before serving.

TIP:

Instead of strawberries, which are only available fresh for a short time, you could use frozen blueberries or raspberries.

Fabulous fruit cake

SERVES 12
Preparation time: 20 minutes
Cooking time: 1 hour 30 minutes
Each serving provides 197 calories; 24.8g carbohydrate; 4.3g sugars; 8.4g fat;
0.2g salt; 1 portion of fruit.

Ingredients:
75g sultanas
100g raisins
250g candied peel
100ml boiling water
1 banana (about 100g), mashed
2 eggs, beaten
75ml sunflower oil
1 courgette (about 200g), grated
1 apple (about 100g), grated
1 carrot (about 80g), finely grated
150g wholemeal flour
1 tsp baking powder
3 tsp mixed spice
6 glacé cherries (washed to remove syrup)
20g whole blanched almonds

Method:
1. Preheat oven to 170°C/Gas mark 3. Add the sultanas, raisins and peel to a bowl. Cover with the boiling water and set aside.

2. Mix together the mashed banana, eggs and oil in a large bowl and beat well to combine.

3. Mix the courgette, apple and carrot into the banana, then stir in the flour, baking powder and mixed spice. Next add the rehydrated dried fruit, plus the soaking water.

4. Stir to combine thoroughly and put the mixture into a 20cm cake tin lined with baking parchment. Top the mixture with cherries and almonds, cover with foil and bake for 1 hour 30 minutes. Remove the foil 15–20 minutes before the end of the cooking time, then bake uncovered for the remainder of the time, until the top is browned and a knife or skewer inserted into the centre of the cake comes out clean.

5. Leave to cool in the tin for 10 minutes, then turn out onto a wire rack. Invert so that the cherries are on the top again and leave to cool completely.

Carrot and walnut loaf

SERVES 8
Preparation time: 20 minutes
Cooking time: 1 hour, plus 30 minutes cooling
One-eighth of the loaf provides 250 calories; 25g carbohydrate; 4g fibre;
5.8g protein; 5g fat; 7g sugars; 0.2g salt.

Ingredients:
For the cake
300g wholemeal bread flour
1 tsp baking powder
2 tsp mixed spice
1 tsp cinnamon
2 eggs, beaten
1 medium banana, mashed
2 dessertspoons granulated sweetener
50ml rapeseed oil plus 2 tsp to oil the tin
150g sultanas
400g carrots, finely grated
2 tbsp milk

For the topping
250g fat-free cream cheese
1 tbsp granulated sweetener
Zest of 1 orange
20g walnut pieces
Few drops of vanilla essence, to taste

Method:
1. Preheat oven to 180°C/Gas mark 4. Lightly grease a 1lb loaf tin with oil.

2. In a bowl mix flour, baking powder and spice. Add sultanas and grated carrot.

3. In a separate bowl, add eggs and banana and blend well. Add sweetener and oil.

4. Fold banana mixture into dry ingredients. Add milk.

5. Pour mixture into bread tin and bake for 1 hour. Remove from oven and leave to cool.

6. Mix cream cheese with sweetener and vanilla essence in a bowl and spread over cooled cake. Decorate with grated orange zest and walnut pieces.

Red velvet birthday cake

SERVES 24
Preparation time: 40 minutes
Cooking time: 40 minutes
Each 78g slice provides 135 calories; 16g carbohydrate; 3g fibre;
5.4g protein; 5.2g fat; 5g sugars; 0.2g salt.

Ingredients:
200g wholemeal flour
200g plain flour
600g cooked beetroot, blended until smooth
2 tsp baking powder
20g cocoa powder
6 egg whites, beaten until peaks form
2 tsp vanilla extract
5 tbsp granulated sweetener, plus 1 tbsp for the frosting
100ml rapeseed oil
250g quark or fat-free soft cheese
1 tbsp pistachio nuts, chopped

Method:
1. Preheat oven to 180°C/Gas mark 4 and use spray oil to lightly grease a 2-litre cake tin.

2. In a large bowl, mix together the flours, baking powder and cocoa powder. In a separate bowl, beat the egg whites until frothy, then add vanilla extract, rapeseed oil, alternative sweetener and blended beetroot.

3. Stir the mixture into the flour, then fold in half of the egg whites being careful not to knock out the air you've introduced.

4. Pour into the cake tin and bake for 35 minutes until cake feels slightly firm. If it's not firm, leave in the oven for another 5 minutes.

5. Blend the soft cheese and granulated sweetener together in a bowl and set aside.

6. When the cake is completely cool, cover the top with soft cheese frosting and chopped pistachios.

Spicy ginger biscuits

MAKES 24
Preparation time: 10 minutes
Cooking time: 25 minutes
Each biscuit provides 56 calories; 7.1g carbohydrate;
1.3g sugars; 2g fat; 0.1g salt.

Ingredients:
50ml sunflower oil
10g blackstrap molasses
100ml skimmed milk
100g wholemeal flour
1 tsp baking powder
3 tsp powdered ginger
1 tsp mixed spice
8 tsp granulated sugar substitute
1 egg, beaten
1 ripe banana, mashed

Method:

1. Preheat oven to 150°C/Gas mark 2. Place the oil, molasses and milk in a saucepan and heat gently for 2 minutes.

2. Meanwhile, in a bowl, mix together the flour, baking powder, ginger, mixed spice and sweetener. Beat together the egg and mashed banana and add to the bowl with the flour mixture.

3. Line a 30cm baking tray with baking parchment. Gently stir the oil and molasses mixture into the flour mixture and pour into the lined tin (the biscuits will be about 1cm thick). Bake in the centre of the oven for 1 hour, or until the centre of the mixture is firm to the touch.

4. Remove from the oven and leave the biscuit to cool in the tin for 15–20 minutes. Transfer to a chopping board and cut into individual squares.

Sultana and oat tray bake

SERVES 12
Preparation time: 15 minutes
Cooking time: 25 minutes
Each 40g serving provides 130 calories; 15.5g carbohydrate;
4g protein; 5g fat; 5g sugars; 0.1g salt.

Ingredients:
100g reduced fat spread
125g porridge oats
120g wholemeal flour
100ml water
65g sultanas
2 small eggs, beaten
1 tsp mixed spice
1 tsp ginger
1 tsp granulated alternative sweetener

Method:

1. Preheat oven to 180°C/Gas mark 4. Place reduced fat spread in a saucepan and melt over a low heat. Set aside, reserving 2 tsp to grease the baking tray.

2. Mix the oats, flour, mixed spice, ginger and sultanas in a bowl.

3. Add the melted spread and mix, then add the beaten eggs and 100ml of water. Mix well.

4. Grease a 20 x 26cm baking tray with 2 tsp of melted spread. Spoon in the mixture and even out to 1cm thickness.

5. Lightly dust with alternative sweetener and bake for 20-25 minutes.

6. Allow to cool before dividing into twelve pieces and serving.

Savoury cheese scones

MAKES 10
Preparation time: 15 minutes
Cooking time: 20–25 minutes
Each scone provides 113 calories; 14.7g carbohydrate; 0.7g sugars;
3.9g fat; 0.2g salt; ¼ portion of vegetables.

Ingredients:
200g wholemeal flour
1 tsp baking powder
Pinch of white pepper
4 spring onions, chopped finely
75g frozen spinach, defrosted with excess water removed to give 50g
50g low-fat mature Cheddar cheese, grated
½ tsp paprika (optional)
2 tbsp sunflower oil
75ml skimmed milk

Method:
1. Preheat oven to 180°C/Gas mark 4, then place a large baking tray in the oven.

2. Mix the flour, baking powder and pepper together. Add the spinach and spring onion, then sprinkle the grated cheese, reserving 2 teaspoons of cheese for later, into the mixture to distribute it evenly.

3. Make a well in the centre of the mixture and pour in the oil and half the milk. Mix together. Reserve 1 tablespoon of milk for glazing, then add the remaining milk little by little, until you have a soft but firm dough.

4. Lightly flour the work surface and gently roll out the dough until 2cm thick. Cut out the scones with a medium-sized round cutter and place on the hot oven tray. Pull together any scraps of dough and roll out again to get an extra couple of scones.

5. Glaze the tops of the scones with the reserved milk and sprinkle with the reserved cheese, and some paprika if you wish.

6. Bake for 20–25 minutes, until golden brown. Serve warm.

Deliciously quick samosas

SERVES 6
Preparation time: 10 minutes
Cooking time: 5–10 minutes
Two samosas (175g serving) provides 190 calories; 31g carbohydrate;
7.8g fibre; 7g protein; 3.5g fat; 7g sugars; 0.6g salt.

Ingredients:
6 x mini wholemeal tortilla wraps, halved
2 onions, finely chopped
2 cloves garlic, crushed
2 tsp cumin seeds
1 tsp fresh ginger, grated
1 large sweet potato, cut into small cubes
750g frozen mixed vegetables
Spray of oil
Pinch of garam masala, turmeric and sesame seeds
Pinch of chilli flakes
1 tbsp fresh coriander, chopped
Squeeze of lemon juice
Plain flour and water, blended to make a paste

Method:

1. Cut tortilla wraps in half to make into pockets.

2. Spray oil into a frying pan and roast cumin seeds.

3. Place onions, garlic and ginger into a saucepan and heat through until soft.

4. Add cubes of sweet potato and mixed vegetables to the pan, seasoning with chilli flakes, garam masala, turmeric and sesame seeds.

5. Add a splash of water and cover pan with lid. Soften pan contents over a medium heat for 20 minutes.

6. Remove pan lid and add coriander and lemon juice. Allow to cool.

7. Use flour and water paste to seal one side of the open tortilla pocket. Fill each pocket with cooked vegetables and fold in half to seal the other side.

8. Allow the samosas to seal by chilling them in the fridge for 30 minutes.

9. Remove samosas from the fridge and place in oven until golden brown.

Mini onion bhajis

SERVES 25
Preparation time: 10 minutes
Cooking time: 45 minutes
Two mini bhajis provide 42 calories; 5.5g carbohydrate; 1.6g fibre;
2.2g protein; 0.9g fat; 1.5g sugars.

Ingredients:
2 tsp rapeseed oil
400g onions, sliced (peeled weight)
100g chickpea flour
1–2 tsp medium to hot curry powder, to taste
2 heaped tbsp (100g) low-fat plain yoghurt
100ml water
235g peas, mashed
150g spinach
3 sprays of oil

Method:
1. Preheat oven to 200°C/Gas mark 6. Line a baking tray with baking parchment.

2. Heat the onions in a pan with the rapeseed oil for around 20 minutes until soft and turning brown.

3. Place the chickpea flour in a large bowl with the curry powder, yoghurt and water and blend well. Add the mashed peas, onions and spinach, mixing thoroughly, then leave to stand for 5 minutes before mixing again for a final time.

4. Spray some oil on the baking parchment-covered tray and wet your hands before firming the mixture into 25 small balls spaced on the baking tray.

5. Bake on the middle shelf of the oven for 20-25 minutes until golden brown, turning the bhajis after 10 minutes to brown on both sides.

TIP:

You could use low-fat plain yoghurt or crème fraiche blended with some lemon juice and garlic as a dip for these mini bhajis, which make great party, picnic or lunch-box food. These mini bhajis can be frozen individually so they don't stick together and can be reheated at a later date.

Healthy muesli bars

These tasty bars are good for lunch boxes and eating on the go.

MAKES 16 SLICES
Preparation time: 15 minutes
Cooking time: 30–40 minutes
Each 73g bar provides 100 calories; 15.3g carbohydrate; 3g fibre;
2.9g protein; 2.7g fat; 6.4g sugars; 0.01g salt.

Ingredients:
Spray of oil
200g jumbo oats
200ml water
2 small bananas, mashed
2 tbsp granulated sweetener
2 heaped tsp cinnamon
1 medium carrot, grated
1 courgette, grated
1 medium apple, unpeeled and cut into small chunks
100g dried apricots, roughly chopped
50g pumpkin seeds

Method:
1. Preheat oven to 180°C/Gas mark 4. Lightly oil a large baking tray. In a bowl, add oats and water. Stir, then set aside.

2. In a separate bowl, mash bananas to a creamy consistency. Add sweetener and cinnamon.

3. Combine grated carrot and courgette with the banana mixture. Add soaked oats, apricots, apple and seeds and mix well.

4. Spread and press down mixture to 2cm thick on the baking tray.

5. Bake for 30–40 minutes until golden brown. After 20 minutes, check the mixture isn't browning too soon. If so, place a sheet of tinfoil over the baking tray.

6. When cool, divide into 16 slices and serve.

Blackberry and apple delight

MAKES 12 SLICES
Preparation time: 10 minutes
Cooking time: 40 minutes
Each slice provides 156 calories; 17.7g carbohydrate; 7.3g sugars;
7.5g fat; 0.1g salt; 1 portion of fruit.

Ingredients:
100ml sunflower oil
2 apples, cored and grated (skin on)
2 medium eggs
1 tsp vanilla extract
2 level tbsp granulated sweetener
150g wholemeal flour
1 tsp baking powder
150g blackberries

Method:
1. Preheat oven to 180°C/Gas mark 4. Use 1 tsp of the oil to grease a 450g loaf tin.

2. Put the grated apple into a bowl, then add the eggs, vanilla extract, sugar substitute and oil and beat together.

3. Add the flour and baking powder and mix well. Fold in the blackberries.

4. Pour mixture into the prepared loaf tin and bake for 25 minutes until firm and golden and a knife or skewer inserted into the centre comes out clean. Cover with foil after 20 minutes if it's starting to brown too much.

Blueberry and avocado lollies

SERVES 10
Preparation time: 10 minutes
Freezing time: 8 hours
Each 82g lolly provides 78 calories; 8.4g carbohydrate; 1.8g fibre;
1.4g protein; 4.1g fat; 7.6g sugars; 0.01g salt.

Ingredients:
2 small avocados (200g), stones removed
200g frozen blueberries
10 soft dates, pitted
250g milk
2 tbsp lime juice

Method:

1. Place all ingredients in a blender and blend until smooth.

2. Divide the mixture between ten lolly moulds, insert lid and lolly sticks and freeze for 8 hours.

3. Serve straight away or leave frozen until needed.

Spicy orange popcorn

SERVES 10
Preparation time: 5 minutes
Cooking time: 3 minutes
An 18g serving provides 30 calories; 6.2g carbohydrate; 0.2g fibre;
0.8g protein; 0.2g fat; 0.8g sugars; 0.01g salt.

Ingredients:
75g popping corn
1 tbsp olive oil
Juice and zest of 1 orange
1 level tsp powdered ginger
2 level tsp granulated sweetener

Method:

1. Heat the oil in a large pan with a well-fitting lid over a medium heat. Drop in three popcorn kernels. As soon as all three kernels have popped, remove the pan from the heat for exactly 30 seconds. Replace pan on heat and add 50g of popcorn kernels. Replace lid and wait for kernels to pop, shaking gently. Do not remove lid. Once popping has died down, remove from heat and leave for 2 minutes to cool.

2. Place the popped corn into a large bowl and repeat the process with the un-popped corn.

3. In a separate pan, warm the orange juice, ginger and sweetener. Mix and bring to the boil, then continue to heat for 2–3 minutes until the liquid becomes sticky and the volume is reduced.

4. Stir in the orange zest and add the popcorn, mixing well to coat evenly.

5. Spread onto a baking tray and leave to dry.

TIPS:

This popcorn can be put into bags to hand out or served in a bowl at a Halloween party. This recipe also provides a low-sugar alternative to bought popcorn at the cinema.

Useful Contacts

Action on Sugar

Action on Sugar is a group of specialists concerned with sugar and its effects on health. It is successfully working to reach a consensus with the food industry and government over the harmful effects of a high-sugar diet, and to bring about a reduction in the amount of sugar in processed foods.

www.actiononsugar.org

Change 4 Life

Change4Life is a public health programme in England which began in January 2009, run by Public Health England. It is the country's first national social marketing campaign to tackle the causes of obesity.

https://www.nhs.uk/change4life/food-facts/sugar

Public Health England

Aims to protect and improve the nation's health and well-being and to reduce health inequalities. PHE is an executive agency sponsored by the Department of Health and Social Care.

https://www.gov.uk/government/organisations/public-health-england

Sugar Smart UK

Sugar Smart UK is a campaign run by Sustain to help local authorities, businesses, organisations, workplaces and individuals to reduce the amount of sugar consumed.

https://www.sugarsmartuk.org/

Glossary of Terms

Added sugars – sugars added to foods by the manufacturer, cook or consumer.

ADHD – a condition affecting attention, level of activity and impulse control. These difficulties present themselves before the age of seven years and can affect many areas of childhood and family life.

Angina pectoris – a condition marked by severe pain in the chest, often also spreading to the shoulders, arms and neck, owing to an inadequate blood supply to the heart.

Atherosclerosis – a disease of the arteries characterised by the deposition of fatty material (cholesterol) on their inner walls.

Beta-endorphins – a type of polypeptide hormone produced by the brain, especially in the pituitary gland, that blocks the sensation of pain. It is produced in response to pain, exercise and other forms of stress.

Cataracts – an eye condition manifesting as clouding of the lens, impairing vision.

Cirrhosis – a chronic disease of the liver marked by degeneration of cells, inflammation and fibrous thickening of tissue. It is typically a result of alcoholism or hepatitis.

Coronary artery disease – the most common type of heart disease that occurs when the arteries that supply blood to heart muscle become hardened and narrowed. This is due to the build-up of cholesterol and other material, called plaque, on their inner walls, known as atherosclerosis.

Cortisol – a stress hormone that increases blood pressure and supresses the immune system.

Dopamine – a neurotransmitter produced in several areas of the brain. Dopamine is released to support behaviours that are important to survival.

Epinephrine – also known as adrenaline; a hormone that is also used as a medication which causes an increase in heart rate, muscle strength, blood pressure and glucose metabolism.

Free sugars – sugars added to food and drinks such as breakfast cereals, flavoured yoghurts, fizzy drinks, biscuits and chocolate. Additional sugar may be added at home, for example, to cereals, or added during the manufacturing process. Free sugars also describe concentrated sugars occurring in honey and products such as golden or maple syrup, unsweetened fruit or vegetable juices and smoothies.

Fructose – fruit sugar.

Galactose – lactose joined with glucose.

Ghrelin – hormone that stimulates appetite, increases food intake and promotes fat storage.

Glaucoma – a condition where there is increased pressure in the eyeball, causing gradual sight loss.

Glucan – a substance formed from a number of units, also known as a polysaccharide.

Glucose – a simple sugar which is an important energy source in living organisms and is a component of many carbohydrates.

Glycaemic index – a value often assigned to carbohydrate foods based on how quickly or slowly they digest and affect the blood glucose level.

Glycogen (glucose) – a stored form of carbohydrate in the liver and body tissues.

Gout – a painful inflammatory arthritis.

Hereditary Fructose Disorder – a condition causing hypoglycaemia in children because the body can't metabolise natural fruit sugars.

Hyperplasia – an increase in the number of cells in an organ or tissue. These cells appear normal under a microscope and are not malignant, but they may become cancerous.

Hypertrophy – the enlargement of an organ or tissue from the increase in size of its cells.

Hypoglycaemia – low blood glucose caused by too much insulin, strenuous exercise, lack of food or because medication has reduced blood glucose levels.

Insulin resistance – where body cells don't respond efficiently to insulin, meaning blood glucose levels rise.

Lactose – sugar found in milk or dairy produce composed of galactose and glucose subunits.

Lactose intolerance – a common digestive problem where the body is unable to digest lactose, a type of sugar mainly found in milk and dairy products. Symptoms of lactose intolerance usually develop within a few hours of consuming food or drink that contains lactose. Symptoms may include flatulence (wind) and diarrhoea.

Leptin – a hormone produced by the body's fat cells referred to as the 'satiety hormone' or the 'starvation hormone'. It regulates fat storage so that in times of famine, the body has an energy source by using stored fat.

Macular degeneration – a condition where the central part of the retina at the back of the eye deteriorates.

Maltitol – a sugar alcohol also considered to be a carbohydrate that is found in some fruits and vegetables. Sugar alcohols are sweet, but not quite as sweet as sugar, and have almost half the calories.

Maltose – a sugar produced by the breakdown of starch by enzymes found in malt and saliva. It is a disaccharide consisting of two linked glucose units.

Microcrystalline cellulose – a term for refined wood pulp and used as a texturiser, an anti-caking agent, a fat substitute, an emulsifier, an extender, and a bulking agent in food production. The most common form is used in vitamin supplements or tablets.

NutraSweet – an artificial sweetener made from aspartame.

Oestrogen – the primary female sex hormone. It is responsible for the development and regulation of the female reproductive system and secondary sex characteristics.

Peripheral vascular disease – a blood circulation disorder that causes the blood vessels outside of the heart and brain to narrow, block or spasm. This can happen in arteries or veins.

Phenylketonuria – an intolerance to the phenylalanine amino acid found in most proteins. Children with this condition should not be given food and drinks sweetened with aspartame.

Phytoestrogens – plant-derived compounds found in a wide variety of foods, most notably soy. These compounds have many health benefits such as reducing the risk of osteoporosis, heart disease, breast cancer and menopausal symptoms.

Polycystic ovary syndrome (PCOS) – a set of symptoms due to elevated androgens – male hormones – in females. Symptoms of PCOS include irregular or no menstrual periods, heavy periods, excess body and facial hair, acne, pelvic pain, difficulty getting pregnant, and patches of thick, darker, velvety skin.

Pre-diabetes – also known as insulin resistance – defined as blood glucose concentrations higher than normal, but lower than established limits for diabetes itself.

Retinopathy – an eye condition describing a number of symptoms including abnormal dilation of the blood vessels in the eyes and bleeds in the retina at the back of the eyes. In advanced cases, the retina becomes heavily scarred and may lead to blindness.

Saccharin – a white, water-soluble artificial sweetener that's 300 times sweeter than sugar. Often used by people who want to lose weight or who must not eat sugar.

Seborrheic dermatitis – a very common skin condition that causes redness, scaly patches and dandruff. It most often affects the scalp, but can also develop in oily areas of the body, such as the face, upper chest and back.

Serotonin – a hormone that gives us a sense of well-being.

Sleep apnoea – a condition where breathing stops for a short time during sleep, caused by a physical closing of the airways. Obstructive sleep apnoea is often found in people who are very overweight.

Sorbitol – a white, water-soluble crystalline alcohol with a sweet taste, found in certain fruits that is metabolised slowly.

Splenda – an artificial sweetener made from sucralose.

Stevia – a plant-based sweetener that combines glucose and steviol.

Sucralose – an artificial sweetener and sugar substitute with no calories as the majority of ingested sucralose is not broken down by the body. Sucralose is about 320 to 1,000 times sweeter than sugar, three times as sweet as both aspartame and acesulfame, and twice as sweet as saccharin.

Sucrose – a compound of cane or beet sugar.

Sugar – a simple carbohydrate that breaks down into glucose in the body.

Sugar Twin – an artificial sweetener made from saccharin.

Sweet'N Low – an artificial sweetener made from saccharin and cyclamate.

Testosterone – the male sex hormone that stimulates the production of sperm in men and the development and maintenance of the appearance of male characteristics.

Total – an artificial sweetener made from aspartame.

Total sugars – all naturally occurring sugars present in the product from sources such as fruit and milk.

Triglycerides – a type of fat (lipid) found in blood. After eating, the body converts any calories it doesn't immediately need into triglycerides. These triglycerides are stored in the body's fat cells where they are later used for energy between meals.

Tryptophan – a chemical used to make the amino acid serotonin.

Type 1 diabetes – a condition caused by auto-immune attack on the insulin-producing cells of the pancreas, resulting in little or no insulin being available to lower blood glucose levels.

Type 2 diabetes – a condition arising from a metabolic syndrome where too much insulin is produced that can't be used to regulate blood glucose levels.

Xylitol – a naturally occurring sugar alcohol found in most plant material, including many fruits and vegetables. It is extracted from birch wood to make medicine and used as a sugar substitute in 'sugar-free' chewing gums, mints, and other sweets.

References

Introduction

[1] *Daily Express* (2 January 2019). 'Children eat 20 stone of sugar by age 10.'
https://www.express.co.uk/news/uk/1066093/children-eating-sweets-sugar-consumption-child-obesity

[2] British Library (1715). A Vindication of Sugars.
https://www.bl.uk/collection-items/a-vindication-of-sugar

[3] Sitwell, K.L. (2017). 'Sugar consumption now vs 100 years ago.'
https://www.linkedin.com/pulse/sugar-consumption-now-vs-100-years-ago-kamila-laura-sitwell/

[4] Yudkin, J. (2012). *Pure, White and Deadly*. London: Penguin Random House UK, p. 13

The Trouble With Sugar

[1] Department of Health (1989). 'Dietary Sugars and Human Disease.' Report on the panel on dietary sugars, 37. London: HMSO

[2] National Diet and Nutrition Survey.
https://assets.publishing.service.gov.uk/government/uploads/system/uploads/attachment_data/file/699241/NDNS_results_years_7_and_8.pdf www.gov.uk

[3] Gardener, H., Moon, Y.P., Rundek, T., et al. (2018). 'Diet soda and sugar sweetened soda consumption in the Northern Manhattan study.' *Current Developmental Nutrition.* https://www.ncbi.nlm.nih.gov/pubmed/29955723

[4] Yudkin, J. (2012). *Pure, White and Deadly.* London: Penguin Random House UK

[5] Jenkins, R. (2018). 'Children eat five times more sugar during summer holidays, study finds.' https://www.independent.co.uk/news/health/children-sugar-consumption-levels-summer-holidays-a8438266.html

Government Action On Sugar

[1] Arthur, R. Watson, E. Michail, N. et al. (18 December 2018). 'Sugar tax: a global picture.' https://www.foodnavigator-latam.com/Article/2019/12/18/Sugar-taxes-The-global-picture-in-2019

[2] Ibid.

[3] IGD (13 August 2019). 'How the sugar tax is changing behaviour.' https://www.igd.com/articles/article-viewer/t/how-the-sugar-tax-is-changing-behaviour/i/22186

[4] NHS (28 February 2018). 'The truth about sweeteners.' https://www.nhs.uk/live-well/eat-well/are-sweeteners-safe/

[5] James, J., Thomas, P., Kerr, D. (2004). 'Preventing childhood obesity by reducing consumption of carbonated drinks: cluster randomised controlled trial.' bmj.com/cgi/content/full/328/7450/1237

[6] Pombo-Rodrigues, S., Hashem, K.M., He Feng, J., et al. (2017). 'Salt and sugar content of breakfast cereals in the UK from 1992–2015.' *Public Health Nutrition* 20(8): 1500–1512

Sugar and Health Issues
[1] Public Health England (2016). *Childhood Obesity Plan for England.* https://assets.publishing.service.gov.uk/government/uploads/system/uploads/attachment_data/file/546588/Childhood_obesity_2016_2_acc.pdf

[2] Health and Social Care Information Centre (2013). National Child Measurement Programme data source, 2012/13. https://digital.nhs.uk/data-and-information/publications/statistical/national-child-measurement-programme/2012-13-school-year

[3] Department of Health (2018). 'Health Survey for England 2017: Adult and Child Obesity.' healthsurvey.hscic.gov.uk/media/78619/HSE17-Adult-Child-BMI-rep.pdf

[4] Health and Social Care Information Centre (2013).

[5] Ibid.

[6] Archer, D. (2014). 'ADHD and refined sugar: can refined sugar trigger ADHD?' https://www.psychologytoday.com/us/blog/reading-between-the-headlines/201404/adhd-and-refined-sugar

[7] Ibid.

[8] Stevens, L. (2019). 'The sugar wars: how food impacts ADHD symptoms.'
https://www.additudemag.com/sugar-diet-nutrition-impact-adhd-symptoms/

[9] Kirchheimer, S. (2003). 'Diet in puberty affects hormone levels.'
https://www.webmd.com/baby/news/20030114/diet-in-puberty-affects-hormone-levels#1

[10] Archer, 'ADHD and refined sugar.'

[11] Papandreoux, P., Karavetian, M., Karaboutai, Z., et al. (2017). 'Obese children with metabolic syndrome have 3 times higher risk to have non-alcoholic fatty liver disease compared with those without metabolic syndrome'. *International Journal of Endocrinology.*
https://www.hindawi.com/journals/ije/2017/2671692/

[12] BBC (3 September, 2019). 'Teenager blind from living off crisps and chips.'
https://www.bbc.co.uk/news/health-49551337

[13] ITV/Rodgers, J. (18 September 2019). 'Mum blames NHS after teenage son goes blind from only eating crisps, chips and chocolate for 16 years.'
https://www.birminghammail.co.uk/news/showbiz-tv/mum-blames-nhs-after-teenage-16932156

[14] Thornton, J. (2018). 'More health warnings on food are needed to reduce tooth decay says BMA.' 360, doi:
https://doi.org/10.1136/bmj.k2177

[15] Srour, B. (2019). 'Sugary drink consumption and risk of cancer: results from NutriNet-Santé cohort study.' British Medical Association.
https://www.bmj.com/content/366/bmj.l2408

[16] Michaud, D.S., Liu, S., Giovannucci, E., et al. (2002). 'Dietary sugar, glycemic load, and pancreatic cancer risk in a prospective study.' *Journal of the National Cancer Institute* 94(17): 1293–1300

[17] Romieu, I., Lazcano-Ponce, E., Sanchez-Zamorano, L.M., et al. (2004). 'Carbohydrates and the risk of breast cancer among Mexican women.' *Cancer Epidemiology and Biomarkers Preview* 13(8): 1283–1289

[18] Franceschi, S., Dal Maso, L., Augustin, L., et al. (2001). 'Dietary glycemic load and colorectal cancer risk.' *Annals of Oncology* 12(2): 173–178

[19] Ibid.

[20] Shama, A., Cantwell, M., Cardwell, C., et al. (2010). 'Maternal Body Mass Index (BMI) and risk of testicular cancer in male offspring: a systematic meta-analysis.' *Cancer Epidemiology* 34(5): 509–515.
https://www.ncbi.nlm.nih.gov/pmc/articles/PMC3069655/

[21] Kirchheimer. 'Diet in puberty affects hormone levels.'

Alternatives To Sugar
[1] Yimaz, S., and Ucar, A. (2014). 'A review of genotoxic and carcinogenic effects of aspartame.' *Cytotechnology* 66(6): 875–881

Planning Low-Sugar Meals

[1] Action on Sugar (2014) 'Sugar in soft drinks.'
www.actiononsugar.org/media/actiononsugar/news-
centre/press-releases-/2016/Fizzy-Drinks-data—2014.pdf

Index